Challenges in Counselling: Loss

Sally Flatteau Taylor

Orders: please contact Bookpoint Ltd, 130 Milton Park, Abingdon, Oxon OX14 4SB. Telephone: (44) 01235 827720. Fax: (44) 01235 400454. Lines are open from 9.00–5.00, Monday to Saturday, with a 24 hour message answering service. You can also order through our website www.hoddereducation.co.uk

If you have any comments to make about this, or any of our other titles, please send them to educationenquiries@hodder.co.uk

British Library Cataloguing in Publication Data

A catalogue record for this title is available from the British Library

ISBN: 978 1 444 1 8772 4

Published 2013

Impression number 10 9 8 7 6 5 4 3 2 1

Year 2016 2015 2014 2013

Cover photo © Yin Yang/iStockphoto.com

Typeset by Datapage (India) Pvt. Ltd.

Printed and bound by CPI Group (UK) Ltd., Croydon, CR0 4YY for Hodder Education, an Hachette UK Company, 338 Euston Road, London, NW1 3BH.

Contents

Preface

There are many books on loss and bereavement/dying and death, and quite a number on counselling people who are facing loss. However, whilst in my work as a counselling practitioner I frequently find myself talking about the wide and varied challenges facing counsellors who are working in loss and bereavement, I've found very few books which focus on this and even fewer which look at ways to face and manage the challenges and enhance counsellors' ability to work with loss and bereavement. This made Kirsten Amis' request to write this book just too exciting to turn down.

The main message from the counsellors I've met is that of not knowing what to say, or how to "be" with bereaved clients. Therefore a main message of this book is that of bereaved people who tell us that they don't need us to have all the answers, but someone who can be truly alongside them, with whom they can develop a supportive relationship and someone who can bear their pain when so many people around them may avoid both them and the subject. They need to be able to explore their issues, sensitive and intimate details of their lives and in this way find the answers and ways of coping for themselves; it's about being rather than doing.

My hope is that as a counsellor or counselling student reading this book it will help you to understand how and possibly why you may at times have a feeling of being out of your depth or out of your comfort zone when working with people facing loss.

Having reflected on this and becoming keen to write this book, I faced a few problems myself during the process and I engaged some of my support network to help me through and I have much to thank them for:

1st: How to identify challenges without the reader feeling overwhelmed and/or deterred from working with people who have been bereaved; to answer this I have tried to make sure that this book can be "dipped into" both from the different challenges and ideas presented, but also from the "management" of anxieties perspective. Colleagues have helped greatly here, especially Jim Kuykendall who has been alongside me as I have developed my practice, and knowledge in loss and bereavement, and who is now moving to work alongside me at The Maypole Project.

2nd: Writing. I have difficulty putting my words onto paper as I frequently have too much to say, which was exacerbated by a strictly limited word count for this textbook. My front line editor, Amanda Taylor, helped me to put things in order and have confidence to complete first drafts.

3rd: Timescale. Having verbally agreed to pick up this gauntlet early in 2012 Kirsten let me know in her usual jocular and persuasive manner that the text had to be completed by December. Wow! – that was something to be considered. However with her support and that of Hodder Education this deadline has been met.

4th problem; during this period we chose to move house, downsizing and moving into a new area was certainly a time of loss for me and certainly added challenge! Parti- David came to the rescue tirelessly packing hundreds of boxes, alongside Mum providing nourishment and occasional use of her spare room to escape to.

5th problem; Maintaining the Maypole Project at a critical time of growth and development was a tough call. Having a brilliant deputy, Nikki Taylor, taking over when necessary helped me and the team through.

So thank you to all of the above for helping me through – thank you most of all as well to the people who have shared their stories with me, and with you.

So as you read on, use this book by scanning the headings and subheadings to reach the areas you need. It cannot due to its brevity cover every possible issue or eventuality, and even as I complete the text I think of more potential challenges and ways to manage them. So I would be really grateful to receive any feedback, and/or any additional issues which you have encountered at sallyflatteautaylor@themaypoleproject.co.uk.

Sally Flatteau Taylor
March 2013

Chapter 1
Introduction

'Between stimulus and response there is a space. In that space is our power to choose our response. In our response lies our growth and our freedom.'

Viktor Frankl

Loss is a large and complex subject; its effects are far ranging and can be likened to the impact of throwing a huge pebble into a pond. After the first impact, which cuts through the calm of the water, its ripples continue to spread across its surface. Loss is an area where no two stories will ever be the same, which is one aspect that I believe makes the work both challenging and fascinating. When we face loss we can't change what has happened – the lost person/object/state of our being will remain lost – but as counsellors we can help people as they face loss, help them as they learn to understand their responses, reactions and coping strategies and, when they feel necessary, find ways to make changes in their responses to such a life-changing event.

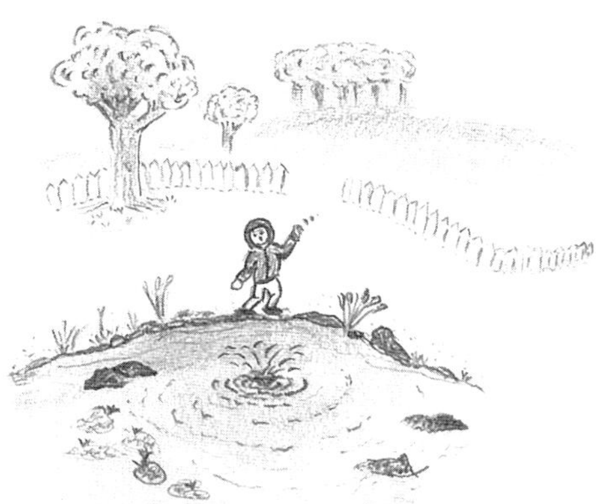

Figure 1.1 Throwing a huge pebble into a pond

This introduction will place the challenges of working with loss into context, take us into the world of loss and **bereavement**, start to define some language around the subject, ask who does this work, why, and moreover why it is challenging.

This chapter will include:

- Entering the world of counselling in loss and bereavement
- Defining some terms
- Who works in loss and bereavement in counselling?
- Why is counselling needed following a death?
- What is a challenge?

Entering the world of counselling in loss and bereavement

As I stepped into counselling training, I found a placement that involved counselling people who were facing loss through death. I felt that I had 'stumbled upon' this placement; however, through training and therapy I quickly realised that I had been supporting people facing loss across many years, talking with bereaved pensioners, and holding an 'open office' morning for pastoral care for staff within my earliest office role. This, followed by multiple experiences of death in my personal life and supporting friends through separation and divorce, gave me an initial insight into the breadth of the issues in loss. Bringing my own background experiences into the present helped me to understand how I didn't stumble upon but actually walked into working in loss and bereavement. Today this still helps me to identify boundaries around the subject so that I neither consciously nor unconsciously merge or overlay my experiences onto my bereaved clients.

My placement at 'The Bereavement Centre' led to: assisting in its development; creating a volunteer support team; training in various settings; and supervising. In 2003 I founded The Maypole Project, supporting families who have children with **complex medical needs** through the losses they encounter from the child's diagnosis onwards, providing face-to-face counselling and support across South East London and nationally via a telephone helpline and providing support services for allied professionals.

As Maypole was born, I became Chair of the Association of Bereavement Service Co-ordinators (ABSCo), a **specialist** network for bereavement support professionals in hospices and palliative care. Most recently, in response to expressed need for training, I founded LACES – Loss Across Consultancy, Education and Support. My work has involved me in counselling people with a wide range of presenting issues, with supervision of counsellors and students, with training and consultancy, reviewing and developing bereavement services. My ongoing studies have led me to researching clients' perspectives of counselling following a loss. These experiences, the places I have been and the people I have met have all informed the content of this book. One aspect I found I quickly needed to learn was an understanding of the language of loss, some terms of which are defined below.

Defining some terms

Loss is losing something we are attached to. This can be loss of a person (through death, which is the focus of this book), of an object, or of our 'being'.

One of the joys of human nature is that we can love. We form attachments to people, to objects and we are also attached to our being; our being can be our levels of ability, our age and stage of life. When you consider this aspect of humanity, it becomes easier to understand that loss will be an integral and inevitable element of life. For a diagrammatic representation of loss highlighting its breadth see Figure 1.2 below.

When we have lost something, we are in the state of bereavement, experiencing the state of loss. On bereavement we grieve or mourn; we go onto a rollercoaster of emotions and feelings. The 'jargon' of loss and bereavement/counselling will be highlighted in bold in the text and explained more fully in the Glossary.

We also need to look at who carries out this work.

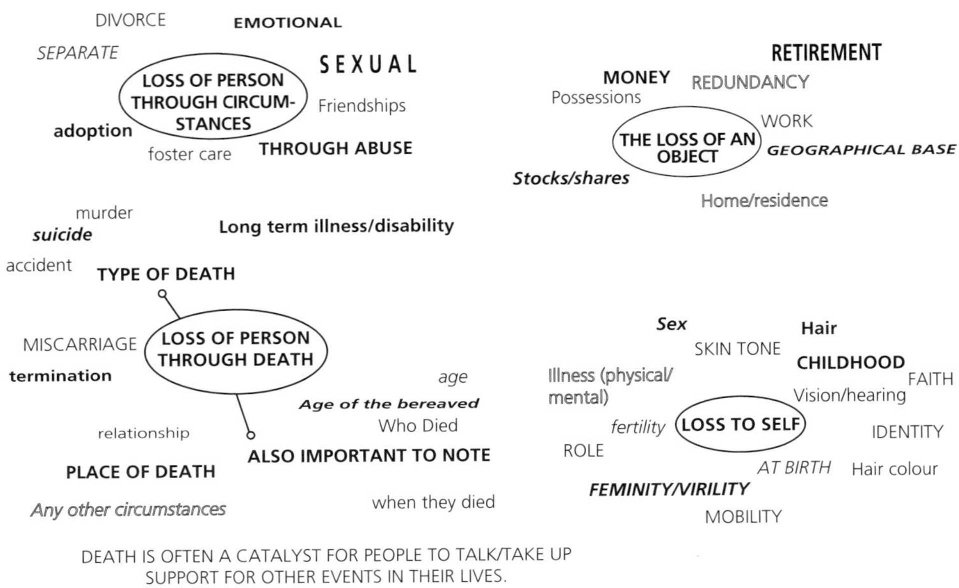

Figure 1.2 The dimensions of loss

Who works in loss and bereavement in counselling?

Counselling for people facing loss and bereavement can be provided through a specialist counselling service. However, loss is an experience which affects everyone, so it is an issue which most clients present with wherever they access counselling.

When I started asking for feedback for this book it was reflected in the range of responses I received from counsellors who were not in a specialist setting.

I noted 'bookend' reactions from:

> *'Loss is central to my work, central to life and life experiences of my clients.'*

to:

> *'A client who I find has faced a loss in their life? I refer them to the specialist service.'*

The different texts on that bookshelf will be explored through this text. However, the difference in response may emerge from an exploration of the meaning of roles.

Counsellors who specialise in working with people facing loss often say they are carrying out **bereavement** or **grief counselling**. This can be defined as counselling which aims to help people cope with grief and **mourning** following the death of loved ones, inferring that the counsellors will support people about the loss in their life. However, loss impacts on every area of one's life: physical, biological, social, economic, mental, and linguistic; it has an **holistic** impact. The root of the word holism is ὅλος (holos), a Greek word meaning all, whole, entire, total. This is the idea that all aspects of a given cannot be determined or explained by its component parts; this has a really good 'fit' with loss and bereavement. If the impact affects all of life, it will require an holistic response from counsellors. The fact is that all counsellors work with loss all of the time, and prefer to re-name a specialist counsellor as one who 'works with bereaved people'. In order to be holistic practitioners we need to have some understanding of all aspects of loss and how it affects a bereaved client's life and being.

Why is counselling needed following a death?

The following sections note that there is a need to counsel people facing loss through death, and it creates challenges and stressors for bereaved people which are outlined in Chapter 4. How this affects us when we are counselling is the focus of this book.

Here I outline four main reasons why such a high percentage of clients bring issues surrounding loss to counselling sessions.

Natural communities of support are less available

Society's response to death has changed across the years, which has resulted in the former natural communities of support being less accessible. Society has moved from the public displays of grief in Victorian times, when graveyards were places where grief was demonstrated through large romantic headstones. Queen Victoria made grief acceptable when she demonstrated mourning publicly at the death of Prince Albert. Following the two World Wars, with the **trauma** of mass death, both death and dying became depersonalised. With the development of the Welfare State came increasing numbers of hospitals and, when treatment failed, dying in hospital made death more invisible and private (Aries, 1981). In parallel with this, society became geographically spread as families moved apart from each other. Graveyards, often local and therefore easily accessible, serving local populations, have given way to increasing numbers of large and less accessible crematoria.

Lost for words

A central theme with bereaved clients is their difficulty in talking about experiences of death to friends and acquaintances. They describe how people 'cross the road' to avoid talking to them, or avoid the subject. This reflects a difficulty in society in facing death and the level of taboo which exists today.

A loss will turn your life 'upside down'

Loss can be a life-shattering event and an experience which can and will provoke a series of powerful emotions that can create a ripple effect into surrounding relationships and activities. Much more can be affected than the loss itself, which can leave people feeling they are struggling to cope; coping mechanisms that may have worked before may not work now.

Varying reactions to different types of loss

Reactions can be affected by different factors of loss such as the type and strength of relationship the bereaved individual had with the deceased. This will be affected by the age and/or stage of life of the person who has died, or the way in which he or she died. For example, the experiences of sudden and violent deaths are often highlighted as being more problematic for clients.

What is a challenge?

I have at times found my role quite challenging, not least because the stories brought to me by clients, supervisees and students raise many complex issues. I have also met many fellow counsellors and allied professionals who acknowledge the level of challenge we can experience both personally and professionally when we work with loss and bereavement.

A challenge can present us with stress, a natural human condition in which we respond to change. It can be positive and manageable, leading to growth, or negative, distressing, uncontrollable, overwhelming and then destructive (Selye, 1976).

Selye also notes that we can cope by resolving our responses, exacerbate the problem through non-resolution, or actively seek a resolution. It is the last-mentioned that we aim to promote within this book.

Losses are identified as among life's highest challenges/stressors, with death taking the lead. So whenever we counsel bereaved people we are counselling stressed people and, in parallel, we can run the risk of becoming stressed ourselves.

It is important to acknowledge that in order to motivate ourselves, we need a certain level of challenge and stress to remain healthy; if we work through the challenges then we will grow both personally and professionally. Only when challenge and stress are at too high a level and remain there for too long can we go into overload and possibly burn out. This text highlights how important it is to 'get it right' both for counsellors and their clients.

The aim of this book is to create a resource for counsellors in practice; whether this is in a specialist setting, as an element of the general counselling we provide, or whether we are yet to qualify. The book will also provide some insight for professionals from other disciplines who meet and support bereaved people.

The starting point is always to 'name' those challenges: the issues that we face that can cause us some anxiety. The next step is to put this into the context of our practice; then to note some ways in which we can manage the issues, by checking whether how we cope now is working for us and creating new coping mechanisms where necessary.

The aim is to notice the level of challenge/stress we are facing, so that we can alleviate it either before we reach a 'plateau', or before this high level of stress is held for so long that we reach 'burnout'. The objectives of this book are to identify the issues we face as counsellors working in loss and how we may manage them, so each chapter will focus on a specific anxiety as summarised below.

Issues raised around settings are outlined in Chapter 2, where we have a discussion that considers different settings: specialist **voluntary**

services, departments within a larger voluntary specialist service, a specialist provision within a larger statutory setting, and independent practice. Each setting is explored from the space that is provided, the name of the service, and the job titles within the service. The plethora of issues surrounding the setting of the service impacts on both counsellor and client.

Chapter 3 takes us through the models and theories which are in 'popular' use in counselling today: from stage/phase and task theories through to those which focus on biography, meaning reconstruction, continuing relationships with the deceased, and complications of grief.

Chapter 4 presents some of the anxieties that many counsellors have faced in practice. This chapter will explore the multiple reasons for feelings that 'overwhelm' and other anxieties counsellors face when working with loss.

Strategies for managing our anxieties are outlined in Chapter 5; this includes ways of managing the challenges we face in terms of how loss and bereavement can be integrated into training, supervision, and personal development/therapy, as well as how efficient management can, in turn, help us to manage these anxieties.

Clients' voices can be heard in Chapter 6. This chapter looks at clients' experience of counselling following a loss. Having considered the many anxieties facing counsellors working with loss in previous chapters, it is interesting to identify the anxieties of the clients on entering counselling and their experiences of counselling.

Professional issues are explored in Chapter 7. The issues presented range from the effects that working on loss may have on our employment and employability, through to issues that may arise when working in, or managing, a team. It includes issues about how we present ourselves, publicity materials and how we provide information about the service to clients and fellow professionals. This chapter also looks at quality control through evaluation, monitoring the impacts of our work, accessing appropriate training and supervision, looking at complaints, grievances and whistle blowing.

Chapter 8 focuses on ethical issues in relation to loss and bereavement. The chapter looks at the framework of the BACP Ethical Framework and, in particular, the principles of first doing no harm, honouring the trust placed in us (fidelity), respecting the client's right to be self-directing and promoting the client's well being.

Research in loss and bereavement is ongoing, which is as expected for a subject that is fluid and dynamic and ever changing. Chapter 9 outlines research studies that draw some conclusions about the 'inside' of the counsellor/client relationship and how it could be re-formed. This chapter also looks at some research into specific areas of loss because the mainstream models noted in Chapter 6 are mostly about death as a generic subject and seldom look at specific subjects.

Finally we have a glossary of terms. Language is important in as much as it should not be confusing to us as practitioners, and certainly not to our clients. This section provides an explanation of the terms identified in bold in this book.

This is a 'dip in' text that aims to clearly label issues with accompanying client vignettes/case examples or notes in each area, with pointers to additional reading and resources. It will provide exercises in some chapters to aid reflection on aspects of bereavement. So I would encourage you to dip in and out when different issues arise with clients.

Summary

- It is important to note when working with loss that it is a topic that is all around us. When someone loses a person close to them the individual's whole life can be turned upside down.
- All aspects of life are affected by loss, which make them central to our work. It is also important to acknowledge that loss can create a ripple effect of further losses in someone's life.
- Loss has an holistic impact and therefore requires holistic responses, which is one of the reasons why working with loss is so challenging.
- There are many challenges in counselling people who are facing loss, including the professional and personal anxieties we may have for our client, as well as those we may have for ourselves.
- Above all, it is important to note that however many anxieties you may have about working with loss, or working with loss in the future, you are not alone. Many counsellors find that loss is a highly challenging subject and its effects are multifold. The next chapters will aim to identify some of these anxieties by exploring worries that have affected and continue to affect counsellors who work in this field.

Activity

Each chapter of this book will contain at least one section where we reflect on practice.

This opening chapter presents the themes of the text. Start to think: What has challenged me when working with loss? How have I managed those challenges?

Chapter 2
Settings

'The service (hospice bereavement) . . . it was tucked away. You know what they say "out of sight, out of mind".'

Parent, Flatteau Taylor 2003

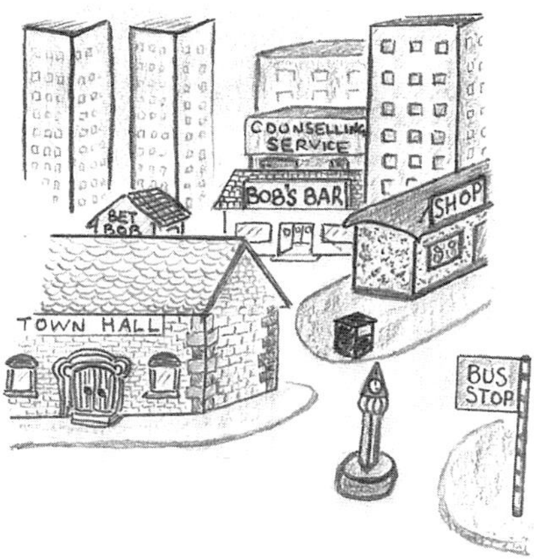

Figure 2.1 The service was tucked away

As counsellors in loss and bereavement we will work in a range of different settings. While there are some guidelines to 'steer' our work in general, they do not appear to identify issues for counsellors when working in different contexts. Each service will have its own specific local cultural differences. What we do find is that within all services the ideal space may be replaced by the most appropriate within funding and local constraints. The aim of this chapter, therefore, is to look at 'setting' in terms of counselling, how different contexts may affect us, in order that we can be prepared for working in these areas. These issues have been identified through personal experience, alongside feedback from colleagues which has provided additional insights, and/or reinforced some aspects. Although the issues are not exclusive to each setting we will look at worries we may find ourselves facing in our counselling practice when we work in the settings outlined below.

This chapter will include:

- **Specialist** voluntary organisations
- Specialism within a broader voluntary setting
- Specialism within a broader statutory setting
- Working independently
- Counselling through an agency, but 'off-site'

Under these headings I have identified issues specifically related to each type of service:

- setting: space and place
- name of the service and associated job titles
- service provision
- line management and supervision.

Note: Other forms of service provision are outside the scope of this book; however, it is important to note that additional forms of counselling such as web-based support, e-counselling and Skype will have their own different contexts.

Specialist voluntary organisations

How does 'specialist' and 'voluntary' affect the setting we are working in?

Setting: space and place

It is a given that the physical place for counselling always needs to be as comfortable, confidential, and accessible as possible. In the voluntary sector, often with the most stringent of budgets, this can be a struggle, but it is possible. The following is a case study of The Maypole Project.

The Maypole Project

Even the smallest room has been turned into a confidential space and used for counselling, with consideration given to what can be heard, and what can be seen in the room from the exterior. Our rooms often have a dual purpose, which is not ideal, but with 'soft' furnishings for the counselling space, clients and counsellors are able to turn their back on the desk/computers. A balance has been reached between safety and the need for confidentiality; for example, where fire doors must have glass panels, obscured glass has been used. Clients of all levels of physical ability need to be able to access the services, but where a building is not suitable for a client, alternatives could be proffered such as home visits (see later in this chapter).

The client's right to accessibility links in with the client's right to privacy and confidentiality. If the agency is clearly marked as a counselling space, consideration should be given to how our clients might feel when they arrive at a service. Do we want to announce 'Bereavement Counselling Here' when clients may prefer a quieter side access door? We explore names further within this chapter.

Comfort is essential. There needs to be as appropriate a level of comfort in setting and space as possible. The setting is the first step for ensuring that the client feels safe and contained. It is important to remember that we are not living in a world where total ideals can be met, but the point is to note the impact of the environment on the client and the counsellor and take steps to minimise any negative effects.

Name of the service and associated job titles

Name

The name of a service can be a message which intends to 'say it all', that is, what you see is what you get. Take, for example, a 'Bereavement Centre'; the name and the focus of the service appear clear: loss through death. Attending a service named 'Bereavement Centre' can also have a profound effect on clients. For some, it means admitting that they need support following a death and suddenly finding they are facing a counsellor for the first time in their life.

Sometimes clients prefer anonymity. However, this can also have an effect on the families attending. 'The Maypole Project' as an agency's name does not describe the service provided, but a leaflet about the services provides a clear description and we still receive enquiries. So is it possible to get a name right? The most important factor is that as counsellors we are clear about what the service provides.

Job title

Counselling in a setting that focuses on loss can mean that we may become identified with that service, sometimes even synonymous with loss and death. This can have the effect that some counsellors steer away from such work. Alternatively, working in specific settings can also infer a level of prestige, resulting in some counsellors being drawn in. This is discussed further in Chapter 7.

Added to this, in the voluntary sector, counselling is frequently offered as a free service and, as such, it is important to reflect on the individual service and what impact this may have on clients. But equally, we need to consider what impact this may have on us as counsellors? We may be extremely pleased to be able to offer a service without charge; we may even feel a little superior!

I am aware that some clients place counsellors on a pedestal; not only are we seen as the 'experts', but we also offer to stay alongside them at a very bleak time in their life. Also, we provide a professional service free of charge. Others may see a free service as inferior; there is no charge, therefore counsellors will be less qualified, less professional and of less value.

Some voluntary organisations, where counselling is free of charge, actively encourage clients to donate and/or fundraise for them. At The Maypole Project we do not promote this, but we find clients still do contribute in some way; sponsored events, for example. The potential impact of this and/or the gifting of any presents should be noted and reflected on as a team and at supervision.

Service provision

The clarity of referral criteria and information given regarding service provision is vital. At The Maypole Project the initial referral criterion was 'children with life-limiting illness/disability', which resulted in some confusion. A professional referred a child who had a limited life as he was deaf; while it is true that deafness may have limited the child's life, it did not meet the rationale that life expectancy would be shortened. We changed the name to 'life shortening'. Subsequently, this has been changed again to 'complex medical needs', as diagnosis and prognosis is not always known and some families therefore did not feel they could access the services.

Clients who are facing loss have noted that their preferred format of counselling provision is through an organisation which uniquely offers that service. They specifically note that when counselling is provided through another discipline (such as a nurse or a social worker) they have held back aspects of their lives.

It is vital that counsellors have an understanding of the service provided so that we can face and support clients with clarity and confidence. This will include not just the type of service that is being provided, but also its boundaries and limitations.

Clients are referred to counselling without an understanding of what it means, and this needs to be explored and clarified before sessions begin. The importance of initial information is also reflected at the end of support; when evaluations are requested the outcome and effectiveness of the intervention can only be measured if the client had known what to expect in the first instance.

It is important to be aware that in developing specialist services we can also be creating exclusive services; this may mean that clients need to move from service to service to access counselling for different aspects of their lives, which can prove very difficult and 'goes against the grain' in a world that is currently strongly advocating inclusion. It would be good practice therefore for services to either keep an information base about different services, or to access such information in order to help clients make informed choices and thus empower them to move to other services as appropriate to them. A similar issue of access applies to counsellors; if we apply to work in a specialist service, would we move 'seamlessly' across services, or would a level of experience and training be required?

In my experience the provision of training within specialist services does hold this tension for counsellors. The majority of specialist loss and bereavement counselling services will insist that any new staff/volunteers undergo their training before they commence working with the service. I have found this to be due to the lack of any standardised training in loss and bereavement and lack of standardised service provision/ways of working (see also Chapter 7).

Line management and supervision

To enable our work as counsellors, it is vital there is clear line management in all service settings, along with effective supervision. However, in smaller independent organisations line management and supervision can, by necessity, be a dual role. The BACP Ethical Guidelines (2010) note the obligation for all counsellors, psychotherapists, supervisors and trainers to receive supervision/consultative support independently of any managerial relationships. However, with separation between the different roles and absolute relationships with the counsellor, this can be managed. Input from external consultants regarding any issues pertinent to this dual role means that such issues cannot only be overcome, but can in fact provide useful additional insight into counsellors' ways of working.

Specialism within a broader voluntary setting

Setting: space and place

Bereavement counselling and support is an element in many broader voluntary service settings, such as hospices and Age UK. However, bereavement services offered as an element of a service provider in the voluntary sector can often be 'tucked around a corner' as unseen and unpublicised provisions. Services provided within a broader setting can feel subsumed under the needs for other areas of support/service provision. For example, the respite/medical services of a hospice will be prioritised over the bereavement support spaces. This could reflect the high level of taboo which remains in society around death and it applies even in organisations that are looking after people in the final stages of their lives. The first example below highlights how important the setting is for our bereaved clients; they felt excluded, pushed out of this service. The second example shows (through lack of space rather than design) how the location of rooms can be more than inappropriate.

Voices

'When my Dad was alive I came to this service through the front door, was welcomed . . . now that he's dead I can still do that, but for support I feel I have to go into a corner of the building – I get a feeling that "out of sight is out of mind" – that is not how I feel about Dad.'

Another bereavement support room was placed alongside the bedrooms in a children's hospice, which caused great discomfort to a number of families; they knew their child would die, but were using the hospice for respite, not end-of-life care and did not want to be reminded of this possibility.

Children's hospices have cold rooms or 'bereavement suites' where a deceased child will 'lay in rest' until a funeral or until the family decide that the child can be taken to the funeral directors. This is an important area for counsellors to be aware of; so too is how the hospice informs staff when a child has died and when a child and their family are using the bereavement suite. It can also be an important element of the care of a child and his or her death.

Name of the service and associated job titles

A service that is an element of a wider voluntary setting may not have a separate service name or identity, as its family support services may, in fact, merge with the wider provision. In 2002, on meeting members of the newly formed Association of Bereavement Service Co-ordinators (ABSCo), I learned of the wide range of titles for bereavement support across hospices' bereavement support workers. This ranged from 'Family Support' to the 'Bereavement Team'. This was an observation which members had different views on, but considering the different cultures in each hospice setting and the difference in the actual roles undertaken, there would probably not be any change in the titles used. The underlying concern of those I met with was the level of experience and training staff had received in order to carry out their role effectively.

Service provision

It is important that when a bereavement service sits within a larger organisation, the assumption is not made that the policies and procedures will fit across all services. For example, bereavement services often need clear and separate referral procedures, as different information may need to be collected and stored (Flatteau Taylor, 2003). Bereaved families do not always wish to return to the place of treatment and/or death so information about other services and subsequent referral should be made available to them, in order that their support remains as seamless as possible at such a difficult time.

Specialist and specific training needs can also become subsumed when a service is provided in a wider context. It is important to be able to access a training provider that will help the team to identify their precise needs and then create a bespoke training package for them. This would include boundaries when working with existing service users who have become bereaved.

Specialism within a broader statutory setting

Setting: space and place

Using working in a hospital as an example, a recent paper by the Department of Health received feedback from 14 or 18 hospital trusts where location was noted (2012). Only three trusts had purpose-built bereavement suites, priding themselves on being in an accessible location for relatives, away from clinical areas. Others noted that the situation of the office was less than ideal, such as the necessity of passing through clinical areas, or long walks noted from the mortuary to the office. Hospital bereavement services tend to centre on more practical issues of support following a death in the hospital setting; for example, helping next of kin deal with the collection of property, guidance regarding what to do after the death, death certification, registration, advice about post-mortems and donation of organs. Sometimes hospital staff will send out routine letters following a death, offering support; some hospitals have counsellors to refer bereaved relatives on, others will refer them to outside external, normally voluntary, agencies (DH, 2012).

Thinking about how clients physically access an area is important. One breast cancer counsellor's office was along the 'service corridor' in the basement of a major hospital, just past the mortuary; this is not ideal. Once inside, however, a room can be appropriately decorated. This needs to be considered in a careful and sensitive manner, as decoration can also have a negative impact. In this case an abstract painting of women's breasts decorated the wall, which had been reported by a client as increasing their distress.

Name of the service and associated job titles

Bereavement officers, nurses with a specialist role, mortuary and pathology staff and chaplaincy are some staff members who generally provide bereavement services within hospitals. They are not necessarily people with counselling qualifications, and while it has been advocated that they should attend courses on loss and bereavement and basic counselling skills to enable them to empathically support families through this difficult period of time, this is not mandatory. Within a hospital setting there will often be counselling/psychology provision, but this is frequently very specialised; for example, women's health counsellors who work with pregnancy loss, still birth, gynaecological issues, cancer counsellors and breast cancer counselling, and so on. The Department of Health's report Bereavement Care Services (DH, 2012) notes that onward referral is frequently made from bereavement officers to voluntary community organisations such as local hospices, a local Cruse branch or local community based support services. Five out of fourteen trusts referred bereaved people directly to their GP, as they felt it was the responsibility of the GP to provide follow-up care.

Service provision

These service providers will be protected and/or limited by the policies and procedures of the hospital setting, but it is important that local policies are created to be specific to the service, just as in larger voluntary settings. Many hospital bereavement services make a proactive offer of support to people whose relatives have died in the hospital setting. They send cards to acknowledge a death, another at around 3 months, and again at 1 year. It has been noted by the Department of Health (2012) that the majority of bereaved families will take up support at 3 months but a proportion also valued the anniversary card and responded at that time. The Department of Health's report identifies that most bereaved people did not pick up services that they were simply 'signposted' to without this active offer.

Working independently

Service providers did not identify any issues specifically related to counselling in loss and bereavement, except for describing an exacerbated feeling of isolation. This will be a theme threading through all counsellors who are in private practice, but when working with clients who face loss and bereavement they can also feel extremely isolated in their lives. This parallel was raised by the practitioners.

Counselling through an agency, but off-site

Within many organisations, counselling is not only provided in on-site counselling rooms, but also off-site. While off-site counselling can be provided by counsellors working for many services, it has been particularly noted in specialist voluntary settings. Taking counselling out of a setting that is within our control may lead to tensions and challenges for a counsellor. It is impossible to list every type of setting but while reading the example below about home visiting, also consider issues that may arise when counselling in other settings such as adult education or in hospital. Although providing very different surroundings these settings will contain similar issues, and there will be issues around the staff within these settings, their understanding of what counsellors provide, and their awareness of the client's need for his or her own private space, perhaps to have some time alone following a session to reflect on the discussion. So let's take a look at some issues which will face us when we provide counselling in a client's home.

Counselling in the home setting

Feedback I have received from many tutors of counselling courses has noted a view that counselling provided in the home is not 'pure' counselling (and often therefore sessions cannot be included in placement hours). However, it is intrinsic to some aspects of loss that home is the only place where such support can be accessed; therefore, we need to be able to meet this need to fulfil our 'duty of care' to our clients. At The Maypole Project we find that our families cannot travel away from home if they have an ill or disabled child who needs constant care. We therefore ensure that we work with them to provide counselling in the setting which is most appropriate to them.

Home visits, meeting with a client in their family's own environment, are also a good way to really learn about a client, as opposed to bringing the individual into a neutral counselling space. However, home visits may also cause more boundary issues, and can be more troublesome for the counsellor than for the client. Such boundary issues may include:

1. *Interruptions*: we cannot control the postman calling or the phone ringing. However, we can create contracts with our clients to minimise these possibilities.
2. *Privacy*: another family member/care staff may be in the home which may cause concerns about confidentiality and may cause constraints for the client who may fear being overheard.
3. *The environment*: we cannot create seating that is set at a comfortable distance apart or on the same level, etc; we have to sit where we can. It is important to check with the client that where we choose to sit is appropriate to them; for example, in case it was a favourite chair of the deceased, or where the ashes are placed.

> **Importance of environment**
>
> A young lady requested counselling after her partner had died suddenly; they had a child with complex medical needs. Entering their living room, I introduced myself and asked where best to sit; she said that I should sit wherever I felt comfortable and I sat on the end of a long, white leather sofa, while she sat on a nearby armchair. After an hour for this first assessment meeting she asked me how I felt sitting where I was. I replied 'very comfortable'. She explained that this sofa was where her husband had slept and where he had died and was reassured when I said that this had not affected me and that I found the space calming.

In brief, specific to loss, visiting people at home following their losses can raise many different issues to be thought through and discussed in training:

- The room; and possessions and photographs of the deceased may be around.
- Ashes are often held in the home.

These objects may sometimes also appear to be a type of 'shrine' of the deceased and may be kept in the client's home. This can be a really important way of memorialising the deceased, providing reassurance with memories, rather than an indicator of complication of pathology in grieving.

When visiting at home we also need to be aware of the need for our own safety. Agencies should have a 'Lone Worker' policy in place and as counsellors we need to ensure that we know this and integrate it into our work, and also use our intuition as well as supervision to monitor any issues.

Summary

- Loss and bereavement counselling is integrated within differing levels across a variety of settings.
- The majority of policies and procedures are created locally; there are few national guidelines.

- However, what does emerge is that loss and bereavement can be seen as a secondary service when it is offered as a part of a wider organisation.
- Whether a service stands alone or is a department in a larger organisation, it will have its own culture and this will always have an effect on the service provided and the clients who receive that service. Some of the impacts are apparent; some are quite hidden.
- The name of the service will have an impact on clients, which we should acknowledge explicitly alongside our job title. It will also have an impact on us as practitioners.
- Working 'off-site' can lead to additional tensions for a counsellor, but can be extremely beneficial for clients due to accessibility of services, being in their own setting and therefore feeling more relaxed and able to talk.

Activity

Create a list of all the settings:

- in which you have provided counselling
- where counselling may be applied.

Consider the issues you have faced or may face, in each setting. Think about the approach of the counselling and how it 'fits' into the service setting.

Further reading

ACT/RCPCH (1997) *A Guide to the Development of Children's Palliative Care Services*. London: ACT (now combined with Children's Hospices UK (CHUK) as Together for Short Lives) and RCPCH.

Available at: **www.togetherforshortlives.org.uk**

DH: The University of Nottingham (2010) Bereavement Care Services: A Synthesis of the Literature.

Available at: **www.dh.gov.uk/en/Publicationsandstatistics/Publications/PublicationsPolicyAndGuidance/DH_123809**

www.bacp.co.uk – British Association of Counselling and Psychotherapy website where you will find branches for counselling in different areas.

Chapter 3
Theory and skills

'She (counsellor) said I had "reached acceptance" . . . then the TV broke down. I miss Steve more and more as time goes on!"

Kirsten (2005)

Knowledge of and understanding theories adds essential information to our work as counsellors. However, there is a balance to be struck between holding a theory as 'the truth' or as 'a truth'; theories which were written as generalisations are turned into directions rather than being used as a 'map' of suggested possibilities in relation to our work with bereaved clients. The importance of holding this tension in awareness is demonstrated in this quote:

> ***'She (her counselor) talked about the stages of my grief, she gave me a book to read about it. I found this quite distressing, my grief didn't seem "normal" then.'***
>
> **Mary in Flatteau Taylor, (2005)**

This chapter aims to provide some background information. Why is counselling needed following a loss? What informs our current understanding of loss and bereavement? It will re-present the major theories in order that we can identify our own 'truths'.

This chapter will include:

- A brief social history: why is counselling needed for bereaved people?
- The foundation of psychotherapy and the beginnings of grief theories
- Early theories of attachment, loss and bereavement
  - Attachment theory
  - Stage theory
  - Task theory
- Critique of earlier theories: a move to the new theories
  - On biography
  - **Dual process model**

- Meaning reconstruction
- Continuing bonds
- Complications in grief
- Counselling theories in loss and bereavement
- A person-centred / integrative approach to loss and bereavement.

- Summary

A brief social history: why is counselling needed for bereaved people?

Loss through death is an inevitable and intrinsic part of life; in past eras people died and were grieved for openly in their community. However, we now live in what could be described as a 'death denying society', where death is invisible, often denied, and taboo (Aries, 1981; Gorer, 1965). Walter (1996) argues that the taboo of death is lessening; it can be seen publicly more now than ever in the news, in high-profile deaths such as that of Diana, Princess of Wales. But does this impact on grief? As a counsellor working with bereaved people, I notice that clients come to counselling simply because they have no one to talk to and, when they do begin to speak, they find themselves having to 'edit' their conversation about the deceased. This difficulty is exacerbated by the way someone has died, and by who has died. These factors can impact on the natural support we receive.

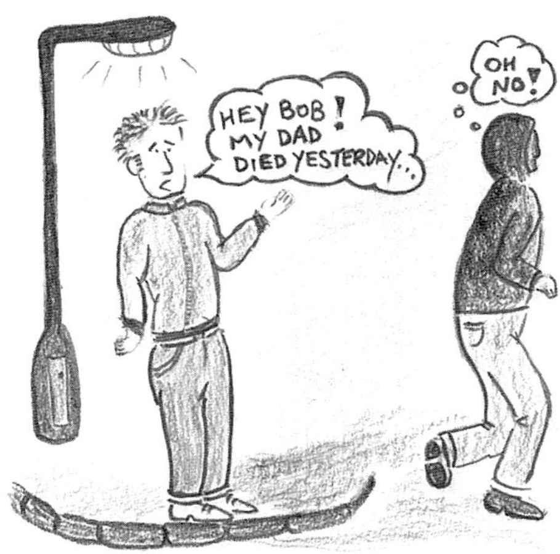

Figure 3.1 Death denying society

Also, while public deaths may be easier to speak about openly, the coverage and conversation can also be at odds with the client's memories and relationship with the deceased, which adds to their angst on bereavement.

In the past, there would also have been more 'natural' support from family who would often be geographically close; there was a greater community spirit and/or stronger attachments to faith groups. In today's world, family members are more distant from each other, often spread apart across countries or continents. There are also different familial patterns forming with increased separation, divorce, and dispersal of members. The world is becoming increasingly secularised, leading to fewer communities of faith. How often do you speak to your neighbours, or attend a community event? I would hazard a guess that in many areas this happens less frequently than in earlier decades.

So with the reduction in traditional methods of support, it appears that there is definitely a need for counselling for bereaved people.

This can be illustrated by research findings in this area. In a report by the Department of Health in 2012 25 per cent of the population were found to need additional support following a bereavement (befriending, mutual help groups) with 7 per cent needing professional support from a counsellor.

These facts and figures highlight that as counsellors we also need to get it right for our clients. Since the beginning of the 20th century, which saw the development of psychotherapy and counselling in the UK, there have been many theorists who have written about the psychological processes of grief. It is important to place these theories into a societal and historical context in an aim to provide some insight into why and how they have developed.

The foundation of psychotherapy and the beginnings of grief theories

The forefather of psychotherapy, Sigmund Freud, described how following a significant loss feelings need to be expressed in 'Trauerbeit' or 'grief work'. He described how the emotional energy of the bereaved needed to be withdrawn from the deceased so that they could then detach from their loss. He outlined that if detachment was not achieved the bereaved person would sink into melancholic depression (Freud, 1917). This became the first influential theory for counselling following a death.

In 1944 Freud's work was incorporated into the research of Lindemann, who outlined stages that would need to be navigated as individuals grieve, focusing on the possibility of mental ill health if feelings were not expressed and detachment from the deceased achieved.

During these formative years for psychotherapy, two World Wars were fought. It is interesting to question whether these world events had any impact upon the development of bereavement theories. Although at this time people were said to 'pull together in the face of loss', the phrase 'stiff upper lip' was popularised in British culture and there was a belief that communities supported each other, the impact of the trauma of war has been noted (Rolls and Chowns, 2011). Just after this period, new thinking was emerging about relationships, bonds, and what happens when an important 'other' dies or is removed from us.

Early theories of attachment, loss, bereavement

Attachment theory

John Bowlby closely studied our patterns of attachment; he suggested that attachment and love would inevitably result in a loss. He noted responses to the loss of a parent; he found expressions of sadness, fear and anger. From this he outlined a paradigm of loss – how people both make and break their affectional bonds (Bowlby, 1969: 80;1979). The way in which people form attachments affects both their grief and how they relate to those they turn to for support throughout their bereavement. It is important to identify in brief the different type of attachments that were outlined at this time.

Secure attachments are formed by children whose parents provided security, sensitivity and were really there for their child(ren). Through this relationship base, separations are seen to be tolerated without anxiety; but this does not prevent strong reaction to sudden/unexpected losses. These individuals will respond well to an opportunity to review their life following significant loss, and often find new meanings in the life ahead.

Anxious/ambivalent relationships are formed by children with parents who were overprotective, anxious and insensitive to their child's need to be independent. The child(ren) may grow up lacking in trust, self-confidence and tending to cling. Separation therefore brings high anxiety. Loss will increase anxiety and clinginess.

Avoidant parents are those who could not express emotions, or closeness. Their children similarly are unable to tolerate closeness and relationship difficulties ensue. Feelings are often not expressed; therefore after a loss, grief may be restrained. Providing a good and safe relationship in support will enable individuals to build trust and express their feelings. An overlying 'gloss' of confidence often hides insecurities.

Disorganised parents are unable to respond consistently to their child(ren)'s needs. Children tend to grow up unhappy, with little trust, feeling helpless. Loss will increase feelings of despair and fear.

It is important to understand a client's attachments, as this can provide an insight into the possibilities of the individual's reaction when an 'important other' is lost. For example, a positive attachment pattern, where primary carers have been attentive and responsive when a baby cries or is fearful, can result in resilience in coping with subsequent losses.

Conversely, insecure attachment or relationships, a lack of comfort or support can mean that feelings have been hidden, subsumed, not expressed; and this can be a factor leading to complications in grief, when a significant loss is encountered later in life (Stroebe and Schut, 2005).

Margaret Ainsworth and S. M. Bell (1970) noted that alongside the psychological responses to bereavement, an understanding of environmental impacts on bereavement was also needed; they noted that each element of a system affects another, a systemic approach.

Stage theory

Through the study of attachment and detachment Bowlby and Parkes defined four stages in the grieving process (1970):

1. Numbness, shock and denial – a sense of unreality
2. Yearning and protest – sadness, crying, anxiety, lack of concentration, guilt, sense of the deceased's presence as a protestation against their death

3. Despair, disorganisation, hopelessness, lowness
4. Re-organisation – letting go of the person who has died.

These stages focus on the psychological processes; they do not allow for an exploration of cultural difference or sociological aspects; they emphasise the resolution of grief as 'letting go'.

Elizabeth Kübler-Ross wrote her seminal work *On Death and Dying* (1969), incorporating and applying Bowlby and Parkes' theories to the process of dying through terminal illness. She slightly changed the stages by adding 'Bargaining' – where patients say 'if only I had' – and changed 're-organisation' to 'acceptance'; the dying person may accept death if he or she is given the opportunity to grieve. The theories of Kübler-Ross are widely taught and can be seen as a basis for theory around anticipatory grief, but are more frequently applied to bereavement following death, rather than dying.

Task theory

In 1981, alongside the swiftly growing profession of psychotherapy and counselling, Worden re-introduced Freud's concept of 'grief work'; he described four tasks of mourning which were:

1. Accepting the reality of the loss
2. Experiencing the pain of grief
3. Adjusting to the environment without the deceased
4. Letting go of the deceased, closure.

It is interesting to note that over the years his defined 'resolution' of grief is one of the most challenged areas in bereavement and this 'task' was amended to 'reinvestment in new relationships' (1991) and to finding an ongoing connection with the deceased while adjusting to life without them (2008).

Critique of the earlier theories – a move to new theories

Through the adoption of these stage and tasks theories it would appear that they have given some support to counsellors working in bereavement. However, it is interesting to note that some authors (Worden, 1981 and Kübler-Ross, 1969) have advocated the use of their theories as 'a' theory rather than 'the' theory, but you will see below and in other chapters of this book that practitioners sometimes do expect their clients to work through stages by completing tasks.

From the 1990s onwards research has increasingly questioned the efficacy of stages and task theories (Haugh, 2001). Craib notes that using stages in bereavement counselling is similar to cutting out gingerbread men – one shape fits all (1994). Stroebe and Schut (2005) notes that there is little scientific evidence to support the idea of stages in grief. In parallel, grief was being re-defined in a broader sense, incorporating sociological, cultural, and anthropological views (Walters, 1996; Rosenblatt, 2001).

Rosenblatt (1993) also notes how, in stepping into someone's world, we need to make sure that our ways of working are not embedded in white western European culture, or the culture of counselling; we need to be able to step into the world and culture of the other.

> 'A sensitivity to cultural differences (such as the wide range of culturally appropriate expression of grief across cultures) should help prevent ethnocentric assumptions that one's own culture or experience necessarily provides a valid baseline for understanding the grief of somebody from a different cultural background. . .'
>
> **Rosenblatt (1993: 104)**

A study of clients' perceptions of counselling (Flatteau Taylor, 2005), which is outlined in more detail in Chapter 9 noted their preference would be to speak about their experiences in their own way.

At its toughest, loss means that we can lose a sense of who we are, our place in the world; this understanding has led to a broadening of our responses from one that focused on the emotional and psychological to that which integrates the vital social, cognitive, cultural and spiritual dimensions of grief. A more holistic approach to loss was advocated as the full impact of a significant death was increasingly appreciated. This gave rise to theories around how bereaved people need to 'relearn the world', after their life was shattered by a significant loss (Attig, 1996).

On biography

Walter (1996) encourages a move away from 'grand theories' towards individualisation of loss as the overarching aim in support. He outlines the bereaved person's need to rewrite the biography of the person who has died, continuing our story about them and about ourselves in the world without them. He emphasises that this can be done naturally in the community without the need for 'outside' support, but where counselling is used, the conversation should be a story about the life and death of the deceased and their transformed relationship.

Dual process model

However, an underlying approach of 'grief work' continued in some theories. A significant paper by Stroebe and Schut (1999) outlined a 'dual process model'. They suggested that although we do need to grieve and the psychological processing of grief is important, we also need diversion; we need to get back to our 'normal' pattern of life. They identify that if we oscillate between grief and diversion this would be normal, but staying on either side of the pendulum would not be helpful.

Meaning reconstruction

Neimeyer (2001) is developing theories around meaningful reconstruction as a central tenet of the process of grief; a social constructivist model. Any major loss upturns our assumptive world, on which our sense of security and expectation of the world is based. Neimeyer concurs with the oscillation process and focuses on the need to continue bonds with the deceased, and reconstruct the meaning of our lives following a loss.

Continuing bonds

In 1999 Klass *et al.* wrote about 'continuing bonds', which underlined how people continue relationships with the deceased through memories, dreams, sense of presence and photographs. In line with Walter (1996) he found that many people have a role in remembering the dead, by creating a narrative around loss, such as friends, family, even pathologists and forensic scientists. He sees the aim of bereavement counselling as helping people to talk about their memories, rather than about detaching from the dead.

Complications in grief

It has been noted that people who are bereaved as the result of unexpected causes, such as violent acts or at a young age, tend to be seen as having 'complicated grief' (CG) (Prigerson *et al.* 1999; Horowitz *et al.* 1997); this was later renamed as prolonged grief disorder (PGD) and it has now been proposed to add this as a diagnostic category in DSM-V (in press, due 2013). Rando (1993) also provides a comprehensive clinical text on the treatment of complicated mourning. However, it is really important that as counsellors we refer our bereaved clients on for a mental health professional to explore such a diagnosis only when, following our own knowledge and intuition in addition to full discussion in supervision, we believe that grief has triggered a mental disorder or restimulated an earlier known mental disorder. When you read DSM IV you will see that many of the presenting issues that highlight potential mental illness can also be seen to be very normal elements of the fluid and dynamic process that we go through when we grieve. Therefore we need to ensure that a client who is grieving, from any form of death, does not become referred inappropriately. In reading these theories you may identify elements which fit your clients' experiences, but I would suggest that no one theory has a total fit. See Chapter 9 for additional research in this field.

Counselling theories in loss and bereavement

Alongside the theories about loss and bereavement, we need to understand the best framework in which to integrate them. Knowledge of family systems and dynamics is important when working with people facing bereavement through death; as the whole structure of a family will change; however, lack of space prohibits exploration here. Psychodynamic theory holds that people have a limit to their levels of emotional, psychological energy that they can invest in relationships, and that following a loss their energy has to be withdrawn to ensure that they can redistribute it into new relationships. The echoes can be heard here of needing to 'let go' of the deceased in order to 'move forward' without them, and re-invest energy in new relationships. Haugh (2011) describes the hold that this 'letting go' hypothesis has in counselling practice, as well as in society as 'breathtaking' and 'deeply embedded'. She further describes it as less than helpful to bereaved people. Psycho Dynamic Therapy also advocates that the impact of loss will take its root from events in childhood.

A person-centred/integrative approach to loss and bereavement

Sheila Haugh (2011) notes the person-centred counselling approach to be most helpful for bereaved people. The person-centred approach is by its nature organismic, about connection and relationship; acknowledging the incredible pain of loss, and helping people to explore why they feel the pain, and how they are coping.

The person-centred counselling approach (Rogers, 1951) is that the client is expert in his or her life and that given the right conditions will find his or her own way forward. The drive to growth and development is a natural human response. The 'right conditions' are the provision of a good-enough relationship with a foundation of empathy, genuineness (congruence) and acceptance (unconditional positive regard). Through this, the person-centred approach advocates non-directivity, accepting their phenomenological experience of themselves, their life and the world.

However, from the client's perspectives an integrative approach is preferred (Flatteau Taylor, 2005). Clients identify the person-centred relationship way of working (non-directive), with some additional attributes that they need from a counsellor. Primarily they need a counsellor who could be more pro-active than traditionally seen in person-centred counselling, although also not overly directive. They want to talk to someone who understands the background of some of the issues they may face, to help normalise their experience when they frequently feel they are out of kilter with the world, and reacting abnormally. Our work as counsellors is not to reassure them, but to be alongside as they put the pieces of their shattered lives back together, albeit this will be in a different shape and pattern. Clients also noted that their primary need is to talk about the loss, the person who had died, their reactions, their extreme angst following the death. Within the foundation of a good relationship, clients found they had an appropriate, safe place in which to explore issues which re-emerged from the past.

It is important to remember that loss through death is an experience of which we are out of control, it is forced upon us, and the only change we can make is through how we react to that change.

Summary

- In the past few decades of psychoanalytical thinking, we can see that there has been a major shift in theory – from the focus on psychological, psychodynamic ways of seeing bereaved people towards person-centred, more holistic approaches.
- More recent theory has a broader focus, integrating differing viewpoints, acknowledging the holistic nature of the experience of grief.
- This chapter provides just an outline of information to give an overview of this shift. It is important to draw on other resources, the additional suggested reading, your own practice, and your own experience to help guide you to the best way of working. It is also important to remember that however many theories you know, each story inevitably will be in some way uniquely different with each client you see, as loss is a unique experience.

Activity

Some theories reflect that loss and bereavement is seen from a psychological perspective; many other disciplines can enhance this understanding.

Think through loss and bereavement from the perspective of different professionals; for example, a sociologist, a doctor, a company manager.

Further reading

Klass, D., Silverman P. and Nickman, S. (eds) (1999) *Continuing Bonds: New Understandings of Grief.* Washington DC: Taylor & Francis.

Stroebe, M., Hansson, R., Stroebe W., and Schut, H. (2001) *Handbook of Bereavement Research: Consequences Coping and Care.* Washington DC: American Psychological Association.

Tolan, J. and Wilkins, P. (2011) *Client Issues in Counselling and Psychotherapy.* London: Sage.

Chapter 4
Identifying anxieties

'No one ever told me that grief felt so like fear.'

C. S. Lewis

This chapter will identify and consider some of the issues we face in counselling practice when we meet a client who has experienced loss through death. It will consider the common worries and concerns that have been highlighted through my counselling practice, in supervision and training; other counsellors working in this area have also contributed their thoughts to this text.

While the language used here will be about 'bereaved people' this is simply for ease of use, and care should be taken not to take an 'objective' view of bereavement; loss affects us all. As loss and bereavement is a uniquely different experience for every person, so it will be for each counsellor; therefore, the ideas listed below cannot be exhaustive. Conversely, it is possible that reading about such a topic may add in some anxieties that may not have occurred to you!

The aim of this chapter is to first contextualise and outline the issues of loss, following the anxieties that have been expressed. Some vignettes are included to 'paint a picture' of these anxieties. Refer to Chapter 5 for ways to manage these issues. Create and maintain your professional and personal resiliance whilst working in this sensitive area.

This chapter will include:

- Facing the issues – loss and bereavement
  - The issues faced on bereavement – placing our anxieties into context
- The breadth of the subject
  - Overwhelm: the ripple effect
  - Death outside of the 'normal' order of life

- Isolation
- The way of death
- Trauma
- Will loss re-stimulate earlier issues?
- Relationship, relationship, relationship
  - Client's relationship with the deceased
  - Counsellor's relationship with the client
  - Counsellor's relationship with self
- Active listening: lost for words
  - Not knowing what to say
  - Client looking for answers
  - Language of loss
- Dealing with strong emotions, and different states of being
  - Sorrow
  - Clients who express suicidal thoughts
  - Fear
  - Anger
  - Relief
  - Guilt
  - Happiness and laughter
  - Non-expression of feeling
  - States of being
- When is grief resolved?
- Summary

Facing the issues: loss and bereavement

Death and bereavement contain multi-layered experiences and responses because it can shatter life as we know it; this makes bereavement a potentially challenging area to work in. To highlight exactly how broad a story of loss can be, this section starts with Figure 4.1, which 'maps' the way in which the process of counselling can be exacerbated when a client has experienced the stress of loss; this is followed by a simple list of some possible experiences that are specific to loss through death.

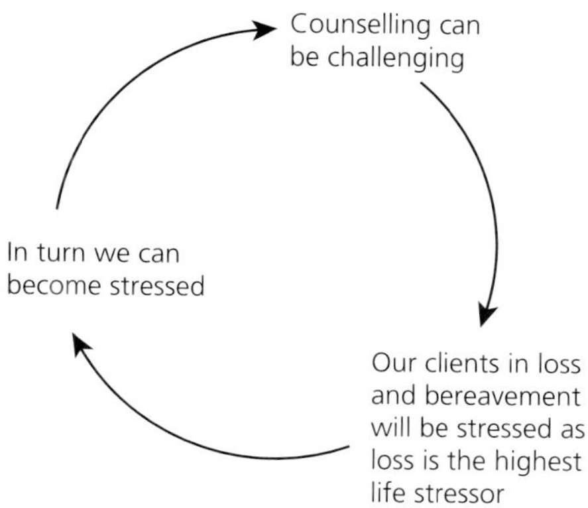

Figure 4.1 The cycle of loss/stress in counselling

Possible experiences specific to loss through death

Different deaths, relationships and co-factors will have a varying impact, for example;

1. Way of death: it may be:
   a expected following a long-term illness (although death may never be truly 'expected')
   b sudden, through short-term illness, murder, manslaughter, suicide (although it is important to note that all death can be sudden even if at some level 'expected').
2. Timing of death/age of deceased:
   a in pregnancy: miscarriage, termination, stillbirth
   b early in life: neonatal deaths, child deaths
   c death of an adult child
   d death in old age
3. It may be a public or private death:
   a death can be public and sometimes high profile due to the type of death (e.g. a gangland murder), or can occur in public, (e.g. road traffic accident), or the death can be made public because the person who died was famous (e.g. Diana, Princess of Wales)
   b death can also be private: hidden in a home, a residential setting, a hospice, a hospital. Death may also be so private that the bereaved become disenfranchised, as others may be unaware of their grief.

Other factors will affect the client's reaction such as:

1. Relationship with the deceased:
   a the person who died will have an impact in terms of their relationship to the bereaved person

   b the death may connect to the bereaved person's role (e.g. vicar's wife/mum to deceased child) and therefore aspects of identity.
2. The age/stage/life experiences of the bereaved person:
   a the bereaved person may react differently due to their age/stage in life, or losses which are earlier, concurrent, or future.
3. Loss through death shatters many aspects of life:
   a role and identity (ties in with relationship)
   b ability to work: finances can be disrupted
   c the security of the home may become threatened.
4. Belief/value/cultures which are questioned and frequently changed.
5. Relationships:
   a the myth that families 'pull together' is often shattered; friends are often 'strangely absent' (although those who were not so close sometimes pull closer); communities are not always there to provide support
   b marital relationships become stressed
   c physical relationships and sex can be affected.

The bereaved will express a range of feelings and reactions: identifying and demystifying the 'ripple effect' of loss:

1. Emotional and behavioural responses:
   a there is a myriad of different responses, from expressing feelings to ways of coping and behaviours.
2. Physical somatised responses such as:
   a fear being present as 'butterflies' in the stomach
   b sense of loss as 'losing half of self'
   c presenting with symptoms similar to the illness of the deceased
   d bodily reactions through repression of emotions, such as
      - stomach upsets
      - heart pains
      - headache.

So what has provoked anxiety? The following themes have been identified during my work with counsellors in supervision and in training, with additional input from colleagues.

The breath of the subject

Overwhelm: the ripple effect

During training, supervision and discussions one of the key anxieties that has been highlighted to me is the enormity of loss.

Voices

Jane, a newly qualified student, remarks on her start of counselling bereaved clients:

> *'What I learnt in training, well that's one thing and this referral seemed quite straightforward, and I knew I was going to be talking about a death. But when it came to meeting the client face to face, I've found her story was much more complicated. I've found it really difficult and a bit overwhelming. Rosie told me about her relationship with her brother, her shock at hearing he had cancer, her chronic sadness when he became ill and then died.'*

Jane continues:

> *'As our relationship deepened, Rosie described how her life had been "blown apart" since his death; in the past, attention from the family had always been on her brother, and since his death her parents had "put him on a complete pedestal", their relationship had disintegrated and she moved away from home.'*

Jane's anxiety was experienced even at this early stage in the client/counsellor relationship; she began to feel that the difference between the theory and the reality was quite overwhelming. Where were the stages she had learnt about at college?

Death outside of the 'normal' order of life

Rosie

Jane was concerned about the dissonance in the family, which she had not expected. Rosie's parents described the death of their son as 'the worst possible thing that could ever happen to anyone', which Rosie experienced as dismissive of her grief, as in her words '*totally unimportant*'. Jane noted the tension she held; needing to really listen to her client and ensure that she valued her story as 'totally important'. Jane had not previously considered different age/relationship to the bereaved in the context of loss and bereavement.

Isolation

Bereaved clients often experience a feeling of isolation, as can be seen through Rosie's story above. They report feeling in a different world, a different culture from others and these feelings can be exacerbated when relationships with friends and family come under stress or even breakdown.

Jane noted how she felt:

> *'. . . quite alone when working with this client; I didn't have the understanding, and I didn't feel I had a supervisor who could help me.'*

So Rosie's sense of isolation raised anxieties for her counsellor; this will be worsened if the counsellor, in parallel with the client, is also feeling isolated in his or her practice.

A further tension held in counselling, arising from the client's expression of feeling isolated can be a fear that the client may become dependent on the counsellor/the counselling relationship (see the section about relationships later in the chapter).

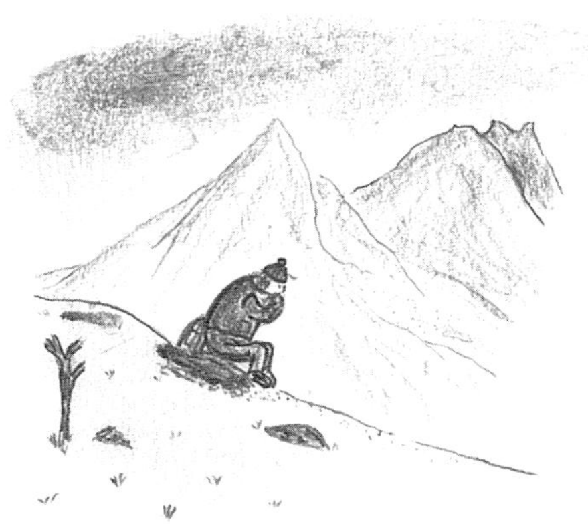

Figure 4.2 Isolation

The way of death

The way a person dies impacts on our clients and, as a result, on counsellors. The way of death can range from long-term illness to violent and sudden death and from public to private deaths. The following are a few brief examples.

Long term illness: cancer

Rosie's brother had died of cancer; Jane's client explored her fear that she may also be diagnosed with the 'Big C'. Was it 'in the family'? She presented with some physical/medical issues, which appeared similar to her brother's. Jane worked on the assumption that this was '**somatised**' illness. However, she expressed anxiety as to whether this was the right way to work. Jane's supervisor advised her to caution – to ensure that her client had checked her physical well being, so that she could continue to work with her through the psychological issues.

Jane's assumption here had been that cancer would mean an expected death which in some way would have been grieved in anticipation, where as she learned that the death came as a shock to the client.

Other long term illnesses and medical fragility may be through degenerative diseases or multiple disabilities.

Sudden death

On receiving a referral, June, a counsellor, reflected her anxiety about the possibility of working with a client who has faced a sudden death.

> *'The referral says that this client's husband had died by "committing suicide" through jumping in front of a train – surely this will be quite complicated, will I be able to work with her?'*

This was June's first experience of working with bereavement by suicide and she had expected to find an anxious client, full of anger and recrimination who would also be full of unanswerable questions, possibly to do with the presence or absence of a suicide note.

Other sudden deaths such as by short acute illness, heart attack, murder or road traffic accident, bring further anxieties for us, as can be seen in the discussion about public deaths below.

Place of death: a public death

A public death can mean: a public place, a public person (famous), a type of death which becomes publicised (a murder). When we see a client who has experienced the public death of someone close there are many issues we face; inquests, post- mortem, and the press, for example. Additional information gained from the press may create a conflict.

'I heard all about how their son died, their wonderful relationship, how everyone came to help. Then I picked up the local paper. The picture was altogether different. What do I do with this additional information?

Sarah, Counsellor (Flatteau Taylor, 2003)

Place of death: a private death

Think about a person dying from a long-term illness cared for at home, in hospital or in a hospice, hidden from public view. This can be most comfortable for bereaved relatives; however, private deaths can also mean disenfranchisement. Friends will not necessarily be aware of the illness or death and therefore cannot care for the bereaved person. Other elements can also exacerbate this. For example, the illness may be one that is hidden from society, such as HIV/AIDS, which continues to have a high level of taboo and will often not be made public until after someone's death; the relationship can be hidden, involving a lover, an unacknowledged same-sex relationship.

Trauma

Counsellors have noted how trauma can be experienced vicariously through the story of their client, as can be seen in the following vignette.

'She opened her purse to show me the pictures of her stillborn child.'

As the counsellor said this to me she shuddered; that body movement said a lot. She described how the photograph had affected her, and she had not wanted to look at it.

We may well be given 'pictures' about loss by our clients. These might be photographs or drawings, which can be very important to the clients. They may also give us a 'picture' through description of the person who has died including how they have died, or an account of an object that has been lost.

When clients chose to reveal such intimacies, how we react will be very significant. They will watch to see just how much of their story we can bear; they will need us to be able to hear everything, to help them explore all aspects of their experiences. The fear of being affected by what we hear or see can become a significant anxiety for counsellors.

Will loss re-stimulate earlier issues?

The following case study was presented in a training session and highlights how earlier issues can be triggered by loss and how these issues made an impact on a student counsellor.

Voices

Becky's grandfather had died from cancer. At the fifth session, she looked down and made a quiet comment:

> *'Granddad did often want me to sit on his lap, I didn't always want to.'*

She explained how she felt her granddad had 'taken liberties' with her after she developed into adolescence. She contained her anger to tell how he had abused her. As he had died she did not want to take any action about this sexual abuse, but she needed to talk about it, her bewilderment at his actions and her responses to him at the time.

The counsellor's anxiety here was experienced in wondering whether this was relevant to bereavement counselling, or whether she had the skills, or should she refer her client to a more specialised service? This was discussed in supervision, and agreed that the counsellor would continue with this client as she worked through the issues of abuse, as it was inter-linked to her granddad, whose death had triggered her memories and given her permission to speak.

Relationship, relationship, relationship

Yes, our relationship with our client is always vital in counselling, but working with loss and bereavement can bring up additional anxieties.

> *'I think my feeling of being overwhelmed may be stopping my ability to empathise and step into the client's world.'*

To empathise, we need to truly step into someone else's world. However, those counsellors and students responding to the question 'What is challenging in working with bereaved clients?' all stated that at times they had experienced difficulties in truly stepping into someone else's world when their experience is a death. Sexton (1999) notes that when starting out, counsellors have felt unable to empathise with people who have traumatic bereavements and that this has resulted in feelings of shame, which they were unable to take to supervision. This, he notes, can result in a downward spiral where the outcome is a lack of appropriate support for the client.

Client's relationship with the deceased

As counsellors we will also hear about a wide range of different relationships; those of the bereaved client with the person who has died and also with the surviving friends and family. In the earlier example, Jane's concern was that Rosie's family appeared to have put her brother on a pedestal, seemingly excluding her. She was concerned about the impact this may have on her client. It is important to remember that whatever the relationship, grief will be individual.

Counsellor's relationship with the client

A counsellor at The Maypole Project noted the potential for anxiety in the client/counsellor relationship.

> *'I am concerned as I am instantly feeling that I will get really drawn into this family.'*

Counsellor, The Maypole Project

Her reasons became clear in supervision and subsequently she used the depth of relationship she felt to ensure that she really connected with a family who had rejected many other services. The relationship became a container for this work and through it she has encouraged and empowered the family to re-engage with other services, so creating a supportive network of professionals around them.

Dependency could have been an issue here. This is often described as a 'no go' in counselling and therapy, occurring both consciously and unconsciously. This case vignette demonstrates how it can be useful as the counselling relationship develops and deepens, as long as we are aware of it (Amis in Dryden and Reeves, 2008).

Counsellor's relationship with self

> *'I've not experienced a close loss . . . will it affect my work?'*

Clients at a bereavement service have frequently asked counsellors whether they have experienced 'the same loss', which has provoked many anxieties for counsellors. It is important to learn how clients feel that this may be helpful to them, while also looking at our own issues. While no two losses are ever the same, nor experienced in the same way, sometimes a similar experience can inform our counselling. However, it is important to note that a similar experience can also hold us back from empathising and truly hearing the client's story, as can be noted in the case study below.

Voices

A student counsellor stated:

> *'I could really empathise; I could really understand what she was going through.'*

On exploration in supervision, this student realised that she was in tune with and responding to her own experience, assuming what the client was feeling, rather than really hearing what was happening for her client.

Personal resonance

We may hear about a death which has particular resonance to ourselves, as illustrated in the following example.

Voices

> *'A caller was a woman of 42, whose 44-year-old husband had died from cancer. He died within 3 weeks of diagnosis. I felt more affected by this call than any others, but why? On reflection I realised the caller was my age, her husband the age of my husband – it could have been me.'*

Sarah, Counsellor

What happens if I face a loss in my life?

This has been a constant concern in my practice. At a time when I may be feeling most vulnerable, such as when facing a personal loss, I need first and foremost to consider my clients and this creates additional tension. When I am grieving myself it may become difficult if not impossible to find the psychological energy to support another. Our overall duty of care is to the client; to ensure that the client is not adversely affected and when, without sufficient insight and support, the dynamics of our counselling relationships even could change to self-support.

Facing our own mortality

Earlier in this chapter we heard from Jane, Rosie's counsellor, who continued to explore her own feelings about this death, particularly the thought that cancer can happen to anyone at any time. Working with loss is a sensitive area, but being with someone in the existential angst of a close death can remind us of our own mortality and the fear that those close to us may become ill or die. These reminders of the fragility of life often bring us to look at our values and beliefs in a parallel process to our clients. In order not to overshadow our counselling these personal reflections should be taken to therapy.

The hope is that if we are aware of the possibilities of experience around loss, we will be aware of (but will not lead the client) to other related issues. Through an exploration of losses and the impact of loss for clients, and simultaneously exploring losses in our own lives, we will be more able to 'keep our feet on the ground' when we work in this area.

Active listening: lost for words

Not knowing what to say

Not knowing what to say, feeling stuck or helpless has been outlined as an anxiety and a challenge when counselling bereaved people. This anxiety has been connected to a feeling of being overwhelmed when the full impacts of loss through death have been realised. On top of this, clients often express a feeling of 'overwhelm' about their loss. Counsellors have said, 'What can I do?' 'Can I say anything that will help?' 'There is no magic wand; we can't bring the dead person back.' Then there's the issue that bereaved people often experience their loss as a taboo; where there is a taboo there may also be an anxiety in speaking freely about the subject, even in counselling. Sometimes this is immediately obvious, but it can start at an unconscious level.

Voices

Judy struggled with a client whose sister had died in a road traffic accident. While feeling that they had explored all aspects of her client's life, the relationship with her deceased sister, the funeral, the subsequent impacts of her death, Judy remained concerned about the high level of anxiety the client expressed. Gradually, she noted that her client had not talked about the death at all. With growing awareness of this, and that it may be a part, if not all, of the difficulty for the client, Judy gently opened the subject of the death in a subsequent session. The client expressed relief at being able to talk about everything, she said:

> *'I didn't want to tell you what had happened, it was so truly horrific.'*

This case study also highlights that clients may, at times, hold back information from us, anxious not to 'hurt' us by telling us all the details, so we may need to be able to give them permission to talk about all aspects of their loss. The language we use can also highlight some difficulties.

Client looking for answers

This is a very common anxiety for counsellors when working in loss and bereavement, as clients are often looking for answers: for example, 'Why did he/she die?' 'Why me?' 'Where are they now they're dead?'

Clients even ask, 'How can you help me? Have you ever had the same experience? I just want her back', resulting in a counsellor wondering 'What can I do? How can I help them, I can't bring back a dead person so what use can I be?' Training and supervision can help us to find ways of responding.

Language of loss

Language is a powerful counselling tool, particularly when dealing with loss; let us take a look at the use of language in three different areas:

- between professionals: terminology/jargon
- in society: which is often cliché or metaphor
- of clients.

Between professionals

As counsellors working in loss, our language can become 'professional jargon'; for example, we could talk about anticipatory, unresolved, or disenfranchised grief. Further definitions of these types of grief are contained in the Glossary. The following is an example of a counsellor expressing anxiety when hearing of another's serious mistake with language.

Voices

'I was told the previous counsellor had described loss to a mother, whose daughter had died, in terms of a theory she had learnt; she said: "loss is like a chair – losing someone is like losing a chair leg, you will have totally lost your stability". The young girl had died from cancer following amputation. The mother quickly ceased the counselling. I felt in fear that I might make a similar mistake.'

Counsellor, Maypole Study, 2005

Counsellors have expressed anxiety in trying to understand and interpret words when used in conversation by professionals. (See the Glossary.) We should also take care not to use the professional jargon when talking to our clients, which we will explore in Chapter 7.

In society

Another noted anxiety is the potential to fall into the use of clichés or to react to the use of clichés such as:

1. On the death of a husband: from one friend to another, 'You'll get over it'.
2. On the loss of a child: from a doctor, 'You're lucky, you've got another child'.
3. On miscarriage: from a friend, 'It's nature's way of telling you that there was something wrong with the baby; it's probably for the best'.

Clients report commonly hearing such phrases. While this book is not specifically about counselling children, it is important to note that counsellors have expressed anxiety when clients have talked about their child's response following a death. Again, language is very significant here.

Voices

A parent attended counselling after her mother had died, and her daughter was having sleep difficulties. She realised that someone had told her child 'your grandma has gone to sleep' and that this description may have been the problem; her daughter feared that if she fell asleep she would die too.

Other phrases we use are that the deceased has 'gone on a journey', 'kicked the bucket', and 'gone to heaven'. These phrases can be equally confusing to both adults and children and possibly reflect a level of taboo of death in society; the avoidance of the words 'dead' and 'dying' is evident.

Of clients

Bereaved clients present challenges to us with their use of language. Frequently, the past tense is used when talking about the deceased but sometimes clients, particularly bereaved parents, will slip into using the present tense and become confused and upset.

Clients may also present us with challenges as they find a language to match their new bleak landscape. For example, 'How do I talk about my family since my daughter has died? "I have two children and hope they don't ask for any more information"; or "I have two children, but one has died". This brings up strong responses from many people, and that, in turn, affects me. I could say "I have one child" but this would be to deny my other daughter has even existed and that doesn't feel right'.

Language may have many different impacts. It appears that we can use words to 'mask' the reality of death or loss, and potentially highlight the taboo of loss in society, for example when we say that someone has been 'lost' or 'slipped away'. This is explored further below.

However, it is important to note that from the client's perspective the way they describe a loss may also be an important coping mechanism. It is really important that, as counsellors, we work carefully with language and choice of expression to ensure that we do not collude with avoidance of saying the words. We should be respectful and, when appropriate in a good relationship, we will be able to open a conversation and potentially challenge their use of words.

Dealing with strong emotions, and different states of being

The array of issues associated with loss may make us start to wonder how indeed we can help; likewise, the range of responses can have the same effect. Bereaved people express feelings of chronic sorrow, anger, and fear. These are what we may expect to see, but they can still raise anxieties for us; then there are issues such as clients who don't show their emotions, and raise the question of can grief be said to be complicated?

Sorrow

Chronic sorrow is often confused with 'depression'; the feelings and states of being on bereavement are very similar to the DSM IV categories for depression. However, most bereaved people feel sad but are not depressed.

Clients who express chronic sorrow and strong emotions can create anxieties for counsellors. We may question whether our client's grief has become complicated, which begs the question, when is grief 'complicated'? While it is important to note that grief is a natural, expected response to a loss, there may also be times when a loss can trigger a mental illness or the re-emergence of pre-existing mental illness. As counsellors we need to take care that we do not pathologise normal grief and take advice from more experienced practitioners when we are in any doubt.

Voices

A counsellor described her sessions with a client whose daughter had died:

> *'Tina is talking about her daughter in the present tense; she doesn't want to talk about her death, or the fact that she is dead, because she feels that she will "go into that pit", as she describes it. I will join her in walking around the edge of the pit; because if she goes there I'm scared that she will become too low, depressed and then suicidal.'*

There is a balance to be gained here – Tina felt that as her counsellor was 'walking around the edge of the pit' with her, she was being well supported and yet the counsellor intuitively felt that the 'pit' should possibly be explored but was anxious that this would take her client 'too low'. This reveals a tightrope between 'being alongside' therapeutically and possibly colluding in an avoidance of talking about death. See also Chapter 6.

Clients who express suicidal thoughts

Listen for expressions such as 'life is just not worth living', and 'why am I going on?' They are very commonly heard from bereaved clients whose lives have been turned upside down after a significant person has died. It is vital in this situation to stay sufficiently grounded so that these comments are not just put on one side or excused because the person is bereaved; it is important not to assume that because of various elements in their life (finance, family around them, etc.) that they will not take any action; remember, you don't know.

During counselling it is important for clients who have experienced a loss to tell their story, to make links in losses and, through this they will also inevitably express their feelings about these life events. While sorrow may be a presumed reaction, people who are experiencing a loss can also express a wide range of emotion. It is important to look at the different feelings which may be expressed, especially those that may make us uncomfortable at times. See Chapter 5 for further exploration in this area.

Fear

Counsellors have reported concerns about their clients' levels of anxiety and how it expresses itself. One counsellor noted, 'Is a fluttering heartbeat an illness or a bodily felt reaction to the loss/fear?' Bereaved clients also talk about having a 'broken heart' and describe pains in their chest, which may signify illness. In these instances it is important to help clients to differentiate between illness and somatised effects of loss (which are common). In parallel with any counselling we provide, it is important to ensure that clients have any physical symptoms medically checked by their GP.

Anger

Anger and death are inextricably linked; this may be a very strong statement, but pause and reflect. If you were bereaved you may be angry:

- that someone you love has died
- at the cause of death: it may be a murder, a road traffic accident, or an illness that could have been prevented

- with your family, following the death (issues around the reading of a will, for example)
- that your belief has not 'held'.

So frequently, when working with bereaved people we are working with angry people. Clients may be angry for any of the reasons above; they may need to talk about this, and express their feelings; therefore, we need to be able to stay grounded in order to help them to express their anger.

Relief

A less reported fact is that people who are facing loss sometimes feel relieved; for example, someone dies after a long illness, a separation after a traumatic relationship, or finally a diagnosis after a long period of illness without explanation.

Voices

> *'I thought he'd gone off, found another woman, my deepest nightmare . . . I was so angry with him. Then one night I lay in bed and looked up the road, I realised he could be there. I became so convinced I called a neighbour. He was; he had killed himself in his van. My first reaction was total relief – he hadn't left me.*

(long silence)

> *You're the first person I've told, it sounds so ridiculous even repeating it.'*

This client's relief soon turned to anger as she had no idea why he had killed himself, and she felt totally abandoned. The counsellor reported an initial feeling of bewilderment and anxiety; she had never previously thought of relief being tied in with loss.

Guilt

Guilt has often been described as anger turned inwards. It is an emotion that has also been described in Elizabeth Kübler-Ross's work on stages (1971) as 'self-questioning' as well as 'bargaining' – 'if only I had/had not

. . .'. While with any generalisation there is a counterview, guilt and loss do appear to go hand in hand and also appear to be almost inextricably linked. This can present an area of difficulty for counsellors, 'How can I shift the client's feelings of guilt? I can see that it is not their fault.'

Happiness and laughter

Not all client sessions are full of tears; there is often laughter too, which can be very therapeutic. Memories can be both sad and happy; if you think about a funeral, for example, there is often a range of stories, with varying emotions alongside.

Voices

'Odd as it may sound, it (counselling) boosted and helped me regain my sense of humour. When the world was very bleak it really helped me cope.'

Bereaved parent, Maypole study (2003)

Non-expression of feelings

Anxiety has been conveyed to me by counsellors when their client does not 'seem to be expressing their grief'. It is important to note that in different cultures, expression of grief will differ; understanding from the client's perspective is essential, and 'not expressing their grief' may be absolutely normal for the individual. Conversely, it is also vital that we don't dismiss strong displays of feelings, as they can be expected and accepted in another culture, and this could be to miss an important indicator in our client's well being.

Alongside strong feelings that may be expressed, there are also different states of being that may be noted when someone is bereaved.

States of being

Death and bereavement also affect people's being, which in turn affects how they feel. For example, in the early days following a loss (however long this may be) people are in shock. This is an impact whether the death is expected or unexpected; sleep patterns are often interrupted and the bereaved person may feel forgetful or out of control.

When is grief resolved?

When working with loss, how do we know when grief is at an end? It is a question I am frequently asked. So can we know when grief is 'resolved'? The simple answer to this can be found in the more recent theories and is that grief does not end. An over-used cliché is that 'time is a great healer'. I would suggest that time does not 'heal', but with time things do change.

As counsellors we need to stay alert to indicators from our clients that demonstrate they may be making some adjustments to their new changed life, such as how they are making (sometimes nearly imperceptible) moves forward, as shown in the following example.

Voices

Mary

Mary's husband died from a heart attack; she entered counselling nine months after his death. She looked very run down; she was exhausted as she was not sleeping well, and was anxious and struggling to cope without him. At the tenth session she started to look brighter and her hair had been done. She had made some new friends and was going out. She also started to feel anxious again, aware that she was changing, beginning to move forward with her life. She said:

> *'It feels like I am on the threshold of a door – if I go through it may feel I've forgotten Tony, then I feel guilty . . . will I forget him?'*

In her closing sessions she realised that she could go out, would still remember him – he would stay beside her.

When Mary's counsellor reported these sessions, she described feeling anxious with her client as she made these changes.

It is important that we take careful note of these indicators, as they could signify issues of dependency of the client: 'If I move forward our sessions will come to an end', followed by 'Don't leave me, I'm not better yet'; or from ourselves as counsellors with a lack of resolution to grief . . . do we feel the need to 'hold on' to our clients until we see that they are better? If so, we could be holding on forever. This is a question which should always be asked throughout counselling and relates to our relationship with our client.

There can be an additional anxiety for counsellors here: the tension between the support we feel our clients need in order to begin to resolve their grief; the thoughts and input of supervisors versus the availability of funding for counselling and the constraints which may be placed upon us by the service we are working with.

Summary

- Loss through death is a multilayered/multifaceted experience, which is uniquely different and will be faced by everyone. A very brief glance has been presented into a wide range of issues of loss, and a similarly brief glance at the challenges and anxieties the issues raise.
- Bereaved people may feel confused, helpless, out of control, overwhelmed and in counselling we may feel this as a parallel process.
- As counsellors we wonder where to start, what to say, how to say it, but the most important aspect is to learn how to meet and 'be' with our clients in their grief, in their story.
- The powerful way in which emotions will be displayed and the state of being of the client can also impact on us and leave us anxious and unsure how to move forward.
- The lack of clearly defined resolution or closure to loss can make us anxious.
- Loss is an ongoing experience and state of being.
- Building a relationship can also be affected. If we are feeling anxious then we need to 'steady' and 'ground' ourselves in order to create and maintain relationships.
- There is a fear that our own personal losses may re-emerge in sessions.
- In parallel with these concerns, counsellors must also personally ready themselves to experience explicit details of a topic that is generally hidden from public view.
- It is also important to highlight the strengths of anxieties as every time I meet a new client, even after years of practice, I still feel slightly anxious; what will they be like, how will they react, and what is their story? If I ever lose that 'scary' feeling then I think it will be time for me to lay aside my counsellor's chair.

- Now we have 'named' our anxieties we need to find, as Selye (1976) notes, ways to 'actively cope' with challenge and stress. Chapter 5 will outline some strategies, techniques and resources that will help to identify coping mechanisms; some specific and some more general.

Activity

Consider the clients you have seen, and the case studies you have read.

How do the ideas presented above meet the anxieties you have experienced? What are the similarities or differences?

Further reading

Dryden, W. and Reeves, A. (eds) (2010) *Key Issues for Counselling in Action*. London: Sage.

Resnick, J. (2004) 'The clinical implications of dependency and counter dependency', *Psychotherapy in Australia*, 10(3): 52–9.

Walter, T. (1999) *On Bereavement: the Culture of Grief*. London: OU Press.

Yalom, I. (1989) *Love's Executioner and Other Tales of Psychotherapy*. London: Penguin.

Chapter 5
Strategies for management of anxieties

'Training? A difficult subject, sensitively handled'

Teacher, Flatteau Taylor, 2003

In Chapter 1 we discussed how we need a certain level of challenge and stress in order to energise us, get us started and keep us going in our day-to-day role and workload. In Chapter 4 we acknowledged that we can and do experience anxieties in counselling bereaved people. We have also recognised that these anxieties appear to be contained in the difference between our preconceptions and the reality when we hear our client's story. To some degree we have also explored why these anxieties exist, while understanding that any issues will differ from person to person. This chapter aims to identify ways and means to help us manage these anxieties. In this context 'managing' does not mean 'erasing'; it is about finding levers to help support us in our work, allay fears and find coping mechanisms to continue counselling and avoid the potential for 'burn out'. The chapter is interwoven with exercises aimed at helping us to reflect on our reactions and our practice; it includes the basic 'needs' in counselling when we look to overcome anxieties and provide the best service we can for our clients.

This chapter will include:

- Training
  - Reflection on practice
  - Issues and reactions in loss and bereavement
  - Looking after yourself

- Supervision
  - Policing and checking boundaries, ethics, policies and responsibilities
  - Teaching
- Personal development
  - Suggested techniques
  - Balance in our lives
  - Johari Window
- Management of practice
- Accessing resources
- Summary

Figure 5.1 links the issues raised as anxieties and challenges to management techniques in training, supervision and personal development.

Training

From my searches there appears to be no counselling training in loss and bereavement at counselling diploma level, as a professional qualification for counsellors. Therefore, in order to prepare ourselves further for working in loss and bereavement additional training is necessary. Figure 5.1 includes some themes for training, and you will note that issues of self-awareness are integrated, as this frequently appears to be the 'missing ingredient' in training programmes about loss and bereavement.

It may be pleasing to note that the process of gaining support has already started! Simply knowing we have experiences in common with others can lessen our fears and feeling of aloneness; creating a 'virtual peer group'. However, the following text will provide more information about these themes, with examples from practice.

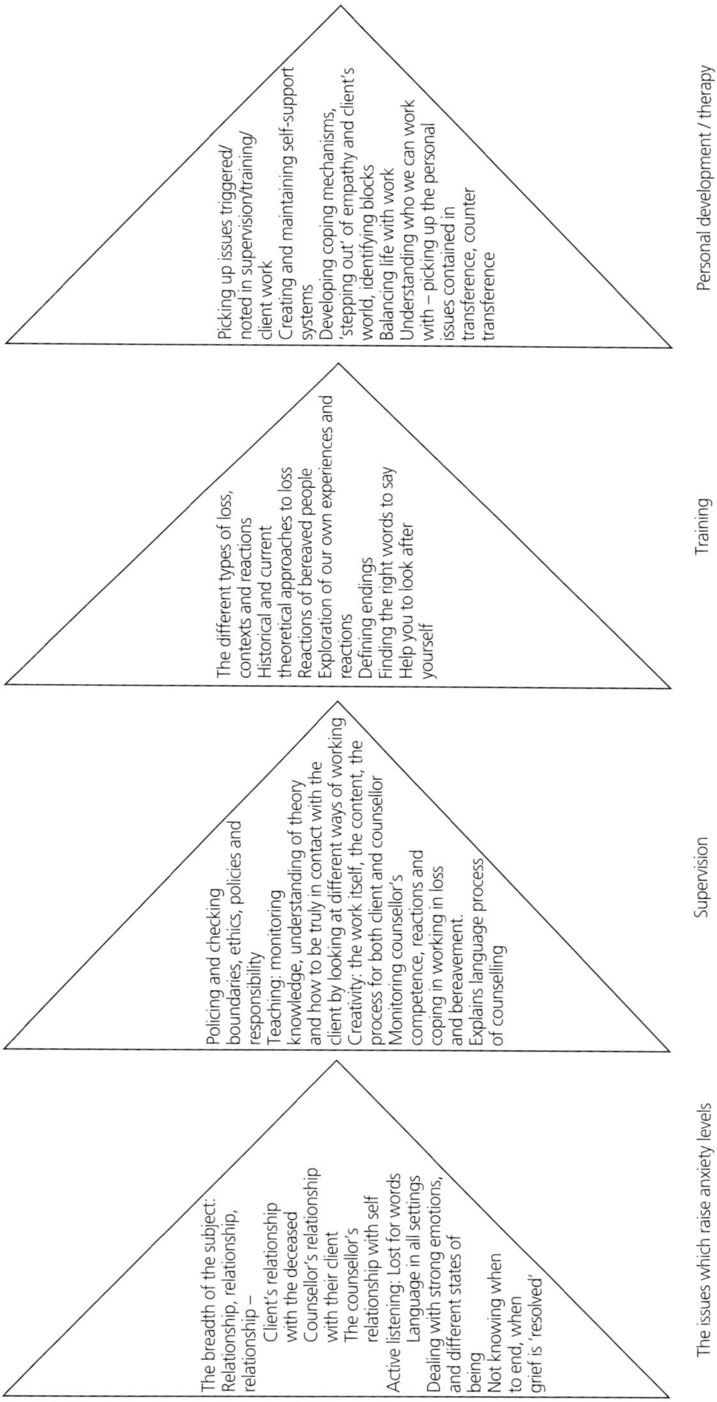

Figure 5.1 Anxieties and management strategies

Issues and reactions in loss and bereavement

Training can alleviate many concerns by simply acknowledging the breadth and scope of loss. A training program should include the following:

- the different types of loss, contexts and reactions
- theoretical approaches to loss
- reactions of bereaved people
- clients who express suicidal thoughts
- finding the right way and words
- defining endings
- exploration of our own experiences and reactions
- looking after ourselves.

Different types of loss/contexts/reactions

When learning about different types of death, the person who died, different contexts, public or private place of death and the shattering ripple effects that death has, it will give us an initial insight into the issues the client may present us with. The parent in the example below notes the importance she placed on meeting someone she felt had a specialist understanding of what she was experiencing.

Voices

'It was important to know that I was really being listened to, and understood, even when I did not particularly understand what I was feeling myself.'

Bereaved parent

Feelings of overwhelm can arise from a lack of knowledge but also through insufficient self-awareness of the issues and their impact on us; therefore a personal exploration of experiences and reactions should be included in training. In order to reach the parts that other courses may not include, loss should be taught in a discursive and experiential way. Examples of some themes, together with exercises are outlined below. Through the course, participants should be encouraged to highlight and explore any specific areas of loss that are particularly challenging to them.

Activity

A young lady was taking a break from dancing outside a nightclub in a city centre when she was sexually assaulted and fatally stabbed; her money and mobile phone were taken. The report of the incident referred to her clothes – short skirt and low top – the fact that she had been drinking heavily, and was outside the club on her own.

What is your reaction to this case?

Think about her age, the fact that she was dancing and the description of her clothes. It would be difficult to read this without painting a picture, and without some personal response.

Theoretical approaches

Up-to-date theories help us to understand the breadth of the subject and the ways of being of bereaved clients. These are explained further in Chapter 6, with on going research the focus of Chapter 9.

Learning about theories will help us to:

- understand the shattering and complicated effects and ramifications of loss
- gain an understanding of how people make sense of their changed lives
- understand how bereaved clients maintain an ongoing relationship with the deceased which helps us not to become anxious if a client senses the presence of the deceased, talks about them in the present tense, or talks of ongoing conversations with them
- understand the importance of relationship between client and counsellor
- understand the need bereaved clients have that their counsellor will be alongside them as they re-tell their story.

When we learn theories, we integrate them into our work, but it is important to use them in the background to inform us, rather than creating a framework of theoretical meaning and inserting the client.

Table 5.1 below outlines some questions that you can ask yourself to find out whether you have a framework around loss and grief. We all have our own values and beliefs and we should test them regularly. Give yourself time to think these through, and allow time for a reflection to follow.

Activity

Some questions about loss, bereavement and grief are posed in Table 5.1. Answer the questions now by circling your response. Refer back to this questionnaire at a later date to see whether your values and beliefs have changed in working with clients and reading this book.

Table 5.1 Questioning our values and beliefs about loss and bereavement

Question/statement	**Response**			
How long does grief last?	3 months	6 months	1 year	Forever
Children grieve			True	False
Children should go to funerals			Yes	No
Death of a child is harder to bear than the death of an adult			Yes	No
How a person dies has an impact on grief			True	False
Grief can lay unresolved and can re-emerge years later			True	False
Children and adults are naturally resilient to loss			True	False
Families pull together in the face of loss			True	False
Loss through death strengthens an individual's faith and belief			True	False

Reactions on bereavement

On meeting clients in their strange new world of bereavement, we will often experience strong emotions and strong reactions from them, which, in turn, can bring up some powerful responses from us. Working with strong emotions has been expressed as an anxiety by counsellors. Training should help us to understand the range of possible responses and help us to explore how we would feel when a client is raging with anger or sobbing in tears. Alternatively, this knowledge could also help us to get inside the world of clients who may not display the type of emotions we might expect.

Clients who express suicidal thoughts

Bereaved people are often very sad and seem very low. It is vital that we take note of any signs that they may be becoming suicidal, without becoming too anxious or reactive. Phrases such as 'life is just not worth living' and 'I'd really like to join him (the deceased)' are frequently used. When appropriate:

- help the client to explore what they mean by those statements
- explore for any specific intention to take their own life
- consider the support the client has
- explore any previous history of self-harm or suicide attempts
- consider the client's use of medical support (i.e. GP)
- and (if you are not already aware) find out exactly what is making it hard for the client to carry on (don't assume the obvious).

If the client continues to explain that it is just something he or she feels, but will not take action, then leave the conversation but do not forget it – use it as a measure for yourself and sometimes it can be used as a measure with clients in sessions. We can use questions such as 'How low are you feeling now, perhaps in comparison with the session when you said . . .'? Always take such client interactions to your supervisor for a second opinion. If you have a sense that your client has underlying feelings that are stronger than he or she speaks of, it is important that you ask direct questions. Some counsellors have noted difficulties in this area (Reeves *et al.*, 2004). Through these questions, make sure that your exploration is deep and thorough and take it immediately to your supervisor or through channels appropriate to your service guidelines. Should your client say that he or she has the means to take their life in hand and has taken steps to plan doing so, it is important to follow guidelines but also be aware that the overriding need is for action to be taken as soon as possible. Ensure that you always have an emergency contact number to hand for your service in case of any such occasion. Such limitations to confidentiality should be included in pre-counselling contracting and the contract re-negotiated at this time to ensure that your client is aware if you need to break confidentiality. And you should identify five key people services your client may contact, should he or she feel very low at times when unable to contact you.

Keeping our feet on the ground and not becoming over-anxious are the most important factors when counselling people expressing strong emotions. Because of this, some 'grounding' techniques are mentioned below.

Activity

Think of a client you have seen recently:

- What emotions did he or she express?
- How did you facilitate the expression of emotions?
- Is there anything which would hold you back?

Figure 5.2 provides a picture-guide to the development of counselling sessions in parallel to the development and deepening of a counselling relationship. It is shown as a 'dip' but in truth will be made up of several dips, looking more like a rollercoaster. However, diagrammatically it does give some pointers to the deconstructive elements of counselling when a client is telling us their story and opening up issues. At this point the client may feel extremely vulnerable and the anxieties we experience may also be at their height.

At the reconstructive stage the client may appear more robust; however, the process continues potentially with a change in patterns of reactions, as the client makes adjustments to life. Paradoxically, this time is fraught with additional losses – leaving old ways of being and taking on the new. We need to be aware of this, and the fact that this can be a time when clients may feel more dependent on our support. It is also important to remember that 'reconstruction' will mean different things to different people – for some clients this may not fit at all. Think through language and include 'adjusting', 'adapting' and 'living with the loss'. (See also Chapter 2.)

Finding the right ways and words

The themes of the issues outlined are:

- not being able to respond
- feeling 'speechless'
- worrying about finding the right words
- being able to empathise with clients who are presenting difficult stories and strong emotions.

It is important therefore to develop a counselling skills framework for our work with clients who are facing loss and bereavement.

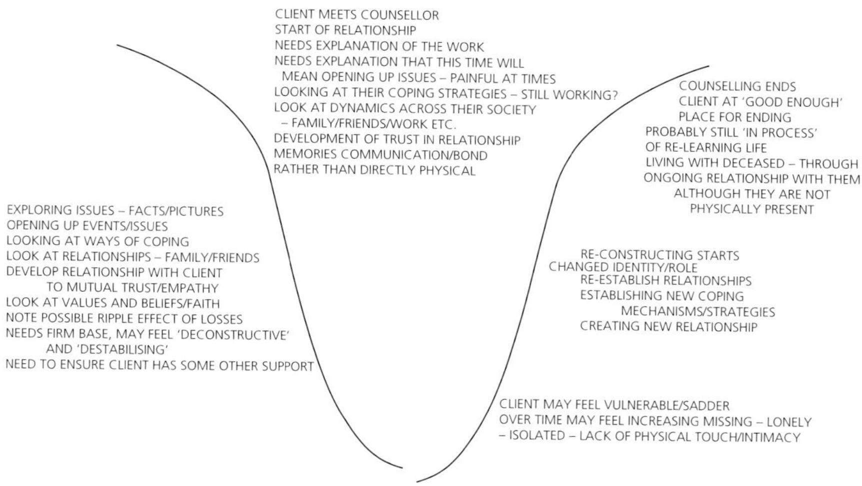

Figure 5.2 The process of counselling following a loss

Research has identified that the foremost important element to counselling for clients has been the relational aspect or the 'being' of their counsellor, as opposed to what they do or say. Rogers (1951) notes empathy as stepping into the world of the other, which is often described as stepping into someone else's shoes, and we know just how uncomfortable that can be at times, but it is an essential element of the social bridge that we create with our clients. Schmid (2001b) further suggests that empathy is the art of 'not knowing'. The overriding need, I would therefore suggest, is for counsellors to be able to listen and truly hear clients' stories in an 'open hearted' way, 'not knowing' what clients will tell us but being there and waiting to learn from them. The importance of training therefore is to find a programme that not only teaches the full breadth of loss and bereavement, but one that also integrates the raising of personal awareness of our reactions to the subject. In this way, it will provide us with some initial knowledge, which is sufficient to ensure that our ability to empathise and listen is not blocked by our reactions to earlier experiences before we start to counsel.

If we are there to listen and hear, then there are no specific 'right words'; if there were I would have written a script! Rather we need to make sure we are not using the 'wrong words'; using technical 'jargon' with clients, for example, or using theoretical approaches to explain the client's 'stage' or 'task', clichés like 'time is a great healer' or platitudes such as 'you'll get over it'. We know as counsellors that these can be explicitly stated, or sometimes implied – either way they are areas to avoid.

Some words are used to avoid saying 'death' or 'dead'. A deceased person may have been 'lost' or 'passed away'; take care here. We need to be aware that counselling lore would encourage us not to collude with the client by using the same phrases; however, to adjust their language may be to crash through their coping mechanisms. Wording should be noted and challenged when (and if) appropriate and with care and within a strong client/counsellor relationship.

Defining endings

Grief is our response to the loss of someone or something to which we have formed a connection or bond. Loss of this bond can shatter life as it was and we, as counsellors, are there to help the client put things back together again; to find their new 'normal', whatever that looks like. This new state will be unique to each individual. I frequently parallel counselling people following a loss to being a 'loss adjuster' – helping them survey what was there, what has happened, how they feel about what has happened and helping them find ways of putting things back together again. Unlike insurance, we cannot replace a person lost through death, but we can help clients to find strategies to live without the person being physically present. This includes finding ways of coping with everyday issues, expressing feelings, and continuing a relationship with the deceased. This is evident in the theories and research which highlight the lack of resolution to grief in terms of a letting go; it is about moving on but without the dead person.

It is also important to note that any exploration of fears and anxieties is not about protecting or desensitising ourselves when working with loss. It is about increasing our knowledge and awareness of how our fears could affect our relationship with our client, and through this to ensure we are as fully available as possible to our clients. This means hearing their stories, opening our eyes, ears, hearts and intuition to them; holding awareness that their stories of loss will have some similarities to our learning, but may well also be uniquely different.

Looking after yourself

Counsellors need self-care. This can achieved by:

- developing our own coping mechanisms, learning ways of coping and applying them, or finding new ways if the existing methods no longer work
- ensuring that we step out of the client's world at the end of sessions

- transference/counter transference
- boundaries and contextual management of clients
- beginnings and endings – how do we clarify them?
- understanding how able we are to work with clients: What is our current well being? Who am I able to work with?

Supervision

A supervisor is the third corner of a triangle of observation, someone who will look at the process and content of the sessions between client and counsellor. It is important that we have a supervisor who is more experienced than ourselves, and who also has knowledge and understanding of the factors facing clients who have experienced loss (the issue of finding a supervisor is discussed in Chapter 7). Within the foundation of a good-enough relationship as described within the person-centred approach in earlier sections, supervision is a space for:

- policing and checking boundaries, ethics, policies and responsibility
- teaching: monitoring competence, knowledge, understanding of theory and how to be truly in contact with the client by looking at different ways of working
- creativity: the work itself and reflection on practice
- identifying what is said in counselling sessions, the content of the sessions and looking at the process of the sessions with respect to both the client and the counsellor
- working with feelings of overwhelm in counselling and finding ways to cope with them and continue to be in contact with the client.

Voices

Becky noted:

> *'My client, Jo, has just suffered so many losses, I just don't know where to start with him. I feel really stuck.'*

Becky was feeling overwhelmed by the issues of loss presented by her client. Her supervisor helped her to explore ways of identifying and exploring these feelings; she took a sheet of paper and put the issues into bubbles across the page. Finishing her task she re-read the sheet, and found that she could draw lines to link issues, which helped herto realise, firstly, that most issues were 'ripple effects' from the presenting loss and, secondly, that the client had told her of these issues, but not that they were particularly troublesome to her; mostly the feeling of overwhelm was her own issue.

For this client, the presenting issue was her main focus; other life events were not a challenge to her at this time, although they became a challenge for the counsellor. Other clients find that feelings of overwhelm can increase when they make the links between losses, as the realisation dawns that one loss will very seldom be an 'island' – it will be more of an archipelago or a collection of islands.

However, when clients do make these links for themselves they can begin to understand the powerful feelings they are experiencing; bereaved clients report high levels of anxiety, and often say they feel that they are 'going round the twist', as they feel so overwhelmed. It is vital that, as counsellors or students, we explore the possibilities before we start to work with clients to make as sure as possible that we do not experience feelings of being overwhelmed by the subject and neither feel stuck, nor shy away from facilitating the client in his or her exploration.

Policing and checking boundaries, ethics, policies and responsibilities

Through supervision we can make sure that we are aware of, and up to date with, issues such as confidentiality, boundaries, safeguarding, and so on, both in the context of the service/setting of the provision and national/specialist/legal standards and guidelines. This knowledge helps us in our ability to practise – once we have learnt, understood and reflected on these issues, we can put them to one side and be grounded, in order to continue with our counselling practices.

Teaching

The aims of teaching through supervision are to:

- identify the strengths and weaknesses of the counsellor in practice, discovering answers to any dilemmas brought into the supervisory relationship/space and uncovering areas for further study
- to give guidance on aspects brought to the counselling session identifying where it is OK not to know, not to have the answers and not to find the solutions. This is particularly important in counselling

people facing loss where facing the unknown; client's feelings of being out of control and helpless are frequent presenting issues.

Finally, to ensure you get the most out of supervision it is important to stay grounded enough to reflect on the following:

- how you are feeling in relation to your client
- what skills you are using with each individual and how effective you think they are. For example, when working with loss counsellors have reported feeling deskilled. What is it that makes you feel deskilled? It may be the subject matter, but it can also be your relationship with the client
- how you are feeling on a particular day or events in parallel in your life
- any trigger points, any internal 'felt sense' in relation to the client; this may be personal issues that can be highlighted and taken to therapy for further exploration, or concerns with/for the client that can be taken back to a session
- potential parallel processes; the relationship and process between counsellor and supervisor can sometimes be similar to a process between counsellor and client that may have a bearing on the counselling process.

Personal development

In addition to the elements of self-care highlighted above, we also need to ensure that we maintain balance in our personal life, and while supervision will highlight any issues that we may need to revisit in personal therapy, there are other ways in which we can balance life. This equilibrium could be called 'work-life balance' but, in fact, means more to therapists than balancing the usual time at work and time at home in other forms of professional work. This is because personal development and self-care help us to find ways to ground ourselves if we are experiencing difficulty in a session with a client. It is important to remember that sometimes our work also triggers earlier issues which we cannot manage through training or supervision, and re-entering personal counselling may be the best way forward. This is particularly important when working with loss, because working with clients facing loss in a subculture such as bereavement means:

- There is a scarcity of peer support from other counselling professionals.
- There is a stigma attached to the work you do – you represent loss in a variety of settings.
- You are working with powerful issues which could re-stimulate practitioner issues.

Suggested techniques

Identify your support network. Who is there for you and for which aspects of your life? Fill in the columns shown in Table 5.2 below, and if these headings are not quite right change/amend or add categories.

Table 5.2 Identifying your support network

I need someone who will . . .	At work	In personal life
Listen wholeheartedly		
Understand my world		
Accept me as I am		
Help me come to my own decisions		
Be there for me – whenever		

If you have someone you can reach out to in all settings, you will feel more grounded in yourself.

Balance in our lives

When working in thanatos (death and loss) it is important that we do not become subsumed in this area. We also need eros (love and life) to be present in our lives to create a healthy balance. Figure 5.3 shows a 'wheel of balance', designed by David Brooks (1997) and presented by Jim Kuykendall in training at The Maypole Project in 2012. The centre of the wheel is at 0 and the outer rim at 10 for each section. Fill in your lines and discover what 'shape' your wheel is.

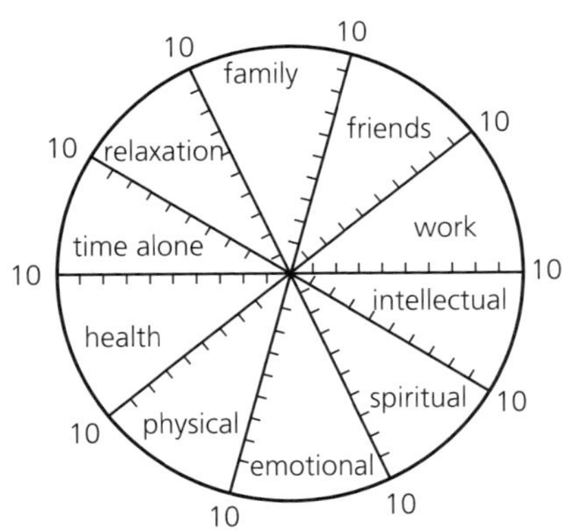

Wheels need to be round if they are to roll smoothly. In the same way our lives need to be balanced if they are to run smoothly; lack of balance can cause distress and/or stress. Take each section and join the lines – where 10 is a lot of time, 5 is enough time and 0 is no time.

Figure 5.3 Wheel of balance

Johari Window

Jo Luft and Harry Ingham (1955) created a model which is now often used to demonstrate aspects of developing self-awareness in counselling.
I find I use this to help clients understand their own level of self-awareness around issues of loss, as well as to explain the process of counselling. The outline given below the figure explains how loss can be used specifically with this model.

	KNOWN TO SELF	UNKNOWN TO SELF
KNOWN TO OTHERS	OPEN	BLIND
UNKNOWN TO OTHERS	HIDDEN	UNKNOWN

Figure 5.4 The Johari Window

1. The OPEN area – is one which is known to the self, and is known by others, the parts of yourself that you are happy with and openly share.

   The aim when looking at the Johari Window is to increase the size of the open window – minimising the others.

Activity

Think of losses past/present and even future which you openly discuss with others:

Who do you discuss them with?
What do you know about them?
How did you cope at the time?
How do you cope now?

2. The HIDDEN area – is known to the self, but hidden from the sight of others. This may be through shame, due to childhood messages which are now out of date for you and unhelpful for growth.

   Self-disclosure will open this area and will only occur in a safe environment/relationship.

Activity

Think of any losses you may have hidden in the past; do you understand why?

May they need exploring in the present to assist with your counselling work?

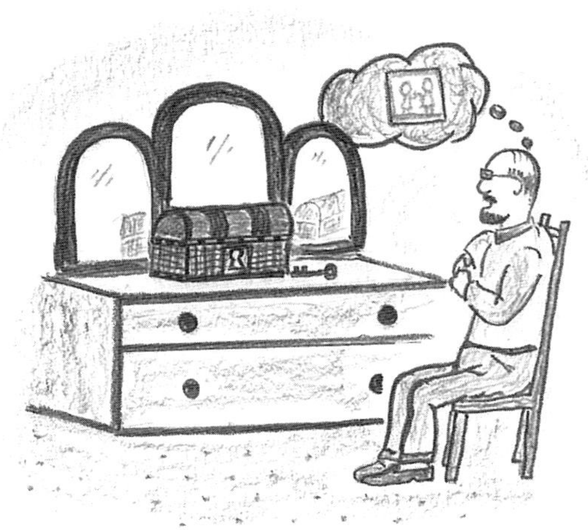

Figure 5.5 Think of any losses hidden in the past

3. The UNKNOWN area; this may be about issues unknown to self, but are more likely to have been forgotten, repressed or denied. Discovering this can be frightening, but also can be exciting.

   Experiment, play, fantasy, myth, story-telling, drama and art can open up this area; and need a very secure relationship base for exploration.

4. And, the BLIND area – unknown to self, out of personal awareness, but others can see them.

   Honest feedback within a safe and supportive relationship, or sometimes play and art therapy will open this area.

These areas are likely to emerge from outside of your consciousness. We cannot predict what we do not recall, but any trigger or recall while counselling should be taken to your supervisor and/or therapist.

Management of practice

Management, or lack of management is shown to provoke anxieties in counsellors. Clear line management and guidelines are vital when working with loss, for example when facing loss in our lives. Policies and procedures should assist if we face a loss or serious issue in our life. It is vital that we consider the impact of personal loss on ourselves, but in parallel this should be taken to discuss and explore in supervision. After that, the issue should be taken immediately to a line manager to check out protocol in this event. It is not always essential, but may be advocated that counsellors take a break through their difficult time, perhaps to return to personal therapy or perhaps to increase supervisory input to ensure that their concurrent loss does not impinge on their ability to counsel. See also Chapter 7.

Accessing resources

Information on brief resources for further training are available in the appendix. It is not an exhaustive list but provides some ideas. Alternatively, conduct an internet search for more local courses and resources, bearing in mind the key attributes noted above.

Summary

- As counsellors we will experience challenges in our daily life; this is not only normal, but also helpful as it both stimulates us in our practice and 'keeps us on our toes' – a bit of 'scary' is good.
- While there are many levers which can help us to manage our anxieties – we will allay them, but we will not necessarily completely obliterate them.
- Managing our anxieties can be about managing expectations: through training we can learn what we *may* expect from clients, their stories, experiences, behaviours, feelings
- We can also start to re-learn and re-think our own experiences and reactions, check that our earlier losses are not re-stimulated in a way in which we are immobilised.
- Through training and supervision we can hear that we don't necessarily need the 'right words'; the 'right way' is best for clients – they want us to be with them and bear their pain and sorrow.

- Through supervision we can explore ways of understanding our feelings of overwhelm; they may be our issue when we hear a client's story, rather than the client's. We can also learn more about specific clients and their unique reactions and way of being.
- In this chapter I have outlined some thought-provoking exercises – do remember that it is also good to discuss these with someone else.
- Find your own networks – local and national – which can provide you with information/support.
- Finally, it can be really important to be aware of other factors that may help you. Having a good resource base of networks, information provision, literature and training can be vital; this text will provide some information, but it is good to expand this with your own local knowledge.

Further reading

Grollman, E. A. (1988) *Suicide, Prevention, Intervention, Postvention.* Boston: Beacon Press.

Schmid, P. F. (2001b) 'The necessary and sufficient conditions of being person-centered: on identity, integrity, integration and differentiation of the paradigm', in Watson, J. *et al.* (eds) *Client-centered and Experiential Psychotherapy in the 21st Century: Advances in Theory, Research and Practice.* Ross-on-Wye: PCCS Books.

Selye, H. (1976) *The Stress of Life* (rev edn). New York: McGraw Hill.

Chapter 6
The voices of clients

'I am afraid to tell you who I am, because, if I tell you who I am, you may not like who I am, and it's all that I have...'

John Powell

The earlier chapters of this book are focused inwards, looking at challenges in our counselling practice from many perspectives. Reflection on our practice is vital, but this chapter demonstrates how important it is listen to, and truly hear, our clients' voices, and this is particularly significant, as Chapter 9 highlights how little research has been carried out in exploring counselling from the bereaved client's perspective.

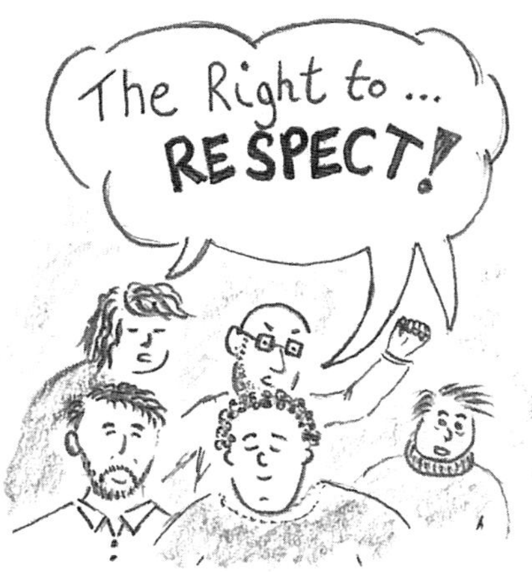

Figure 6.1

This chapter provides the client's stories, and therefore a space where you can compare and contrast the issues each presents to those in the book as a whole. As the quote above reflects, it is important to remember that our clients may have feelings about meeting us. Also as one client noted:

> ***'I've faced a loss; I've never seen a counsellor, never even thought about it, so why now?'***
>
> **Parent, Flatteau Taylor, 2003**

The chapter primarily follows the story of one couple, Tina and Colin, who participated in a study of the experiences of bereaved people (Flatteau Taylor, 2005). The issues faced by this couple mirror the majority of the experiences of bereaved clients we may meet. However, I have added other vignettes, which either run parallel to their experience, or contradict them. Such is the experience of working in loss; no two cases are ever the same.

This chapter will include:

- Presenting Tina and Colin
- Information, information, information
- Right time, right place
  - Setting: 'for people like us'
- Relationship
  - Training
  - The bereaved client's story in counselling: meeting in 'no-man's land'
  - At a time like this
  - . . . Splintered relationships
  - Ongoing relationship
- New languages
  - Language of theories
  - Language in the community
- Feelings: anger, guilt, sadness
  - Power of emotions: 'walking around the rim of despair'
- When does grief end?
- Summary

Presenting Tina and Colin

Their story is outlined here, with actual names and some significant details changed to protect their anonymity.

Tina and Colin

Tina and Colin were teachers. Their eldest daughter Lisa was born with severe medical/learning disabilities; Anna, who is two years younger, has no disabilities. Lisa died at age 13. Their story unfolds throughout this chapter, as we hear about difficulties in their relationships, work, finances and, alongside this, some difficulties in accessing appropriate and effective counselling. They see a psychologist, and three counsellors in two different settings and a mutual help group. Their story has been selected from a study of 12 participants in a study of client experiences of counselling following a significant death (Flatteau Taylor, 2005).

Additional client vignettes are included in this chapter to provide other viewpoints, alongside notes of theories which can be identified.

Information, information, information

Right from Lisa's birth Tina and Colin felt that they needed to talk. Through the hospital they were referred to a clinical psychologist, who gave them a range of information, leaflets and practical advice. They noted a lack of communication about services.

> *'But what is counselling? What is mutual help? How will psychology help us? (. . .) that's what we needed. A guide through the different services, not just leaflets handed out to us. We found it – we had to go looking for it (. . .). It would be so much more difficult for people who are not so receptive.'*

A couple of months after Lisa's death, Tina and Colin knew they needed additional support. At this time, they noticed that hospital staff saw them as a family who could and would cope, which resulted in no onward referral for counselling. They saw the irony of this as they held back their feelings and outward signs of vulnerability in the hospital setting – a place where they felt they had always needed to be seen to be coping and looking after their child and their family.

This links to research that outlines the need for clarity of service provision, from mission statement through to end of counselling, including proactive provision of support (Flatteau Taylor, 2003).

Right time, right place

So, information is the initial key to the door, but for Tina and Colin turning that key to open the door was about finding someone, or some way, to understand individual needs, especially at a time when they felt their lives had been shattered and they were feeling totally shocked:

> *'It is very difficult because to start with you don't even know what you are thinking (. . .) we asked our GP (at 7 months) and he said 'I would give it a bit more time so that you are ready for it' (. . .) for the first three months we just needed each other and Anna.'*

Another national service that Tina and Colin heard about reflected there was '(. . .) a long waiting list, months'. Tina and Colin found this extremely difficult, and they did not access this support as, already feeling out of control and at odds with the world, this wait made things feel worse for them.

Karen and Tom whose daughter died in a road accident, noted the following:

> *'Our GP referred us automatically; the service's policy though was that they wouldn't see people until 3 months after a* bereavement *(. . .) We needed support now.'*

After an initial meeting, counselling was provided fortnightly rather than the weekly appointments that the couple wanted. They said that the counsellor 'gently explained how sometimes the early days are a bit of a "fog" and we may need to miss appointments, due to paperwork, visitors, forgetfulness (. . .). This was hard to hear at the time, but later we realised how right she was, and when we needed more time, there it was straightaway.'

Setting: 'for people like us'

Karen and Tom saw the clinical psychologist a couple of times, but they mentioned that they stopped as they could only see her in hospital. Similarly, when Tina and Colin were referred to a therapist in a hospital setting, Tina made the following comment.

> *'. . . it was even more difficult because we had to go back to the hospital where Lisa had been in intensive care and died – we just didn't want to go back there'.*

The final suggestion came from Tina's Mum who: '. . . found an article about the specialist project – for anybody whose child is ill or has died. (. . .) It was out of our local area, we were not likely to know or meet people in the street outside. We are fairly private about lots of things . (. . .) We could have gone weekly, but we went once a fortnight, it was our choice.'

The centre provided them with support in privacy out of their locality. It gave them a choice of being seen in their centre or at home. A mutual help group was also a distance from their home, and gave them a different type of support:

> *'Later we found The Compassionate Friends (TCF); people's experiences are not the same but similar; we learnt how they've coped and sometimes that helped. It is a meeting of people like us . . . different?'*

This demonstrates how important the right place, at the right time can be; it can provide an essential 'secure base' and good foundation where the work of counselling can flourish. The struggle to achieve this for this family is highlighted here.

Tom and Karen also went to TCF and they noted:

> *'It was very dark, very sad, we lit candles to our children and everyone wore lockets with a picture of their death child. . . not right for us.'*

I have also become aware of how the setting can be an issue for the counsellor, rather than the client. For example, where a service provides counselling to clients who are in-patients in a hospital, unless there is an available side room there is seldom any privacy. As a counsellor this worries me and I ask the staff to respect their patient's privacy. However, this isn't always possible or practicable when medical treatment comes first. Nine times out of ten, clients just want to talk and don't worry who will overhear, as they take responsibility for holding back any specifically private areas until a time when we are in a private space.

This ties into research which outlines that counselling at its best will be offered in the place of choice for the family and, wherever that is, it should be accessible, confidential and comfortable (Flatteau Taylor, 2012).

Relationship

From most theoretical perspectives the relationship we build with our clients is significant, but how do clients see this and what do they want? Tina and Colin identified the type of relationships they have encountered and the effect of each.

They described the clinical psychologist:

> *'She was very pleasant, and it was very practical . . . you could just go and unload but I wasn't getting what I really needed, even though I wasn't sure what this was. I needed someone who could sort of help me find out.'*

They clearly did not want practical help or information without explanation, but this professional was helpful to them as a 'stepping stone' to find effectual counselling.

Of the counsellor at a specialist centre, they said:

> *'She accepted us as very simple people, no judgement on what we chose to do (. . .) no pressure (. . .) very gentle and sort of like everybody's mum, but not motherly nor smothering. We talked through anything and everything; about Lisa, about school (their jobs), about mortgages, how we are coping. What we found really useful (. . .) (is) it is just how you are at the moment, accept how you are today. She helped us see different ways of coping sometimes, because we got very focused on one way of looking at it, can't see anything else. Especially if we were really down or really angry or whatever . . . we just used to get really really tired, chronically tired. . . . she (their counsellor) encouraged us to take Lisa with us as a family (. . .) included in whatever we do.'*

In summary, the important factors for this counselling relationship are that these clients recognised and welcomed a non-judgemental attitude, understanding and empathy, reflecting a person-centred relational base, highlighted by Carl Rogers (1951). They needed a counsellor who would help them to accept themselves, however they were acting/feeling at any time, talk about everything, identify coping mechanisms and help them enhance/change as necessary.

Tom and Karen also appreciated the 'humanness' of their counsellor. They said, 'She was professional, but sometimes people hide behind that don't they – she didn't, she was human.'

Tom and Karen appreciated the honesty of their counsellor about the system and reason for the delay in sessions and her ability to explain the reasons.

Training

Tina said:

> *'I think it makes a difference if people have been trained to work with parents where a child has died, rather than general counselling; they understand some of the issues which we may face, not telling us, just an outline of what may have happened, how we may have reacted. It is really important. The parents I have talked to (. . .) got counselling from the GP surgery (. . .) they do not seem to have thought much of it.'*

This quote touches on training. Tina describes the background information, to help understanding, while in the foreground is the client's story as every client is uniquely different. Tina and Colin found their counsellor's level of understanding most important, her ability to listen and actually hear their story. Other participants in this study noted that they felt dismissed, their story having been deflected, diverted or totally avoided.

Training for counsellors in the specific area of loss and bereavement to enhance self-awareness, thus empathy, has been noted as an essential element in various studies (Flatteau Taylor, 2005).

The bereaved client's story in counselling: meeting in 'no man's land'

The most effective counselling that Tina and Colin experienced following Lisa's death came from a counsellor who helped them initially in talking about their daughter's death, which led them to talk about issues from her life, issues from their earlier lives, and issues for the future. They emphasised how it was Lisa's death that they said they needed to talk about first.

> *'We didn't know what to do (when Lisa died). Are you supposed to be thinking "well that's finished and we have got to start anew"? Is it relief, now for the rest of our lives (. . .)? That wasn't how we felt. We didn't know what was normal or not normal (. . .) we'd been turned upside down.'*

Their daughter's death brought with it strong reactions, emotions, and questions which they needed to express in counselling. They needed to talk about

- her last illness
- her death itself
- how she looked
- how they panicked
- how they wanted her to be at home and how this was an impossibility in the event
- the impact on their surviving child
- their fears and concerns
- that she was now an only child – not the youngest any more, no sibling with disabilities
- the change in their roles – 'we have got to start anew'
- no more caring
- no more forms to fill out
- no more medical teams to meet
- no more appointments
- what does this mean to them?
- what would their world look like now?
- the initial possibility of relief – does this last, will it change?

A change in role means a change in identity as well; parents of children with disabilities frequently agree with Lisa, who described how her identity becomes merged with the child.

> *'People say to me: "Oh, hello, you're Lisa's mum" – rather than "hello Tina".'*

In discussion about these issues around Tina's death in counselling, they also talked about her life, how they were totally shattered at her birth, feeling out of control, thrust into a medical world feeling angry because medicine had not helped them.

Another time they felt:

> *'We were just in no-man's land, didn't know where we were or even who we were any more.'*

The importance to them was that they could talk freely – go from subject to subject without worrying about chronology; the freedom of speech allowed them to reach the corners they needed to talk about. This links to the theory of Thomas Attig (1996), who outlines how bereaved people need to 'relearn their worlds', which have been shattered by death.

At a time like this. . .

As Tina and Colin continued in counselling, their past with Lisa unravelled. They explored how, when Lisa was born they felt they were thrown into a new medicalised world with a new language, new people, isolated and strange and, most importantly, it was neither a world they expected to enter, nor one they had chosen. They explained how they also experienced concurrent losses: issues with family members, friends, problems with work and finances. However, they did not see any of this as loss at the time and they also did not want to look too far into the future; step by step was their motto. As their counselling continued, Tina said they started to explore earlier losses and how she had coped. She explained how she felt upset when issues appeared 'at a time like this', but the counsellor helped them to see that in identifying how they had coped in the past they could either access these coping mechanisms in the present or, if they weren't working so well now, then they could use counselling to consider new ways of coping.

> *'We (Tina and Colin) talked about the past (. . .) when we were ready (. . .) for us there wasn't much to say, our childhood experiences had been good, our families supportive. But we have spoken to other parents whose counsellors have steered them to talk about the past "turning over stones that didn't need to be disturbed"; she said, "I didn't want to go there, I wanted to talk about my daughter". I think that talking about the past can be important, but it's the present that's most important to talk about first.'*

They also noted how their work was affected quite soon after Lisa's birth. They found that they could not concentrate due to the impact of her disabilities. They decreased their hours at work and found they both became carers. 'We only went back part time (. . .) we had lots of support (. . .) when Lisa was ill I gave up full-time teaching for 8 years.' They noted the stress on their finances, the discussions about their roles at home, and their ways of coping had a huge impact on their relationship.

Karen and Tom quickly brought earlier traumas to the surface after their daughter's death, especially some physical problems they had overcome.

> *'When the place burnt down (their company's offices) we were shattered, but we rebuilt the place – and our lives – by taking things step by step, not looking too far ahead, not being too angry about the past – very much living in the day. We got there in the end; spect (sic) we can get there again.'*

Splintered relationships

Tina and Colin experienced problems in sleeping. During Lisa's life she needed 24-hour care and after her death this led to a lack of physical intimacy and exacerbated issues in their marriage. Tina noted how they had pulled away from family and friends, especially where there are young children around.

> *'We have less contact now with family than ever from choice; I don't want to go through pain, watching their pain so it's easier to stay away.'*

She noted how in common with other bereaved families she found that family and friends did not always support them and noted how families can 'splinter' as a result of loss.

Ongoing relationship

Both Tina and Colin continued their relationship with Lisa as they felt her within them; they had ongoing conversations about her, often talking about her in the present tense, talking to her pictures around the house and also through sensing her presence.

Tina said:

> *'When my babies were little, you know they just sort of sat here (demonstrating a baby lying on her tummy) – that's where I feel Lisa is, it's sort of physical . . . I breathe her in almost.'*
>
> *'She loved bubble bath . . . one of the last things she had in hospital was a bubble bath, so (after her death) I found it really difficult to go into the bath . . . Then one afternoon I thought "I'll have a bath" . . . and as I was drying myself I heard her and felt her, felt her presence there . . . "I've enjoyed my bath, mum, I'm going now". It was like she was going home; it was such a sense of relief that she was actually choosing to go.'*

Colin added:

> *'That changed you. . . I came home that day, just totally different, relieved and relaxed.'*

Tina's sensed presence of her daughter brought the new message that she had chosen to leave this time.

It is important to note that for some people a sense of presence of the deceased can be less positive, but the exploration of the subject was vital to them.

As with many bereaved people, mementos, photographs, clothes, and bags were really important to Tina and Colin.

Tina and Colin said they:

> *'. . . give us the feeling of taking our child with us, keeping her in our lives, even though she's not physically here.'*

Similarly, if there has been a cremation, families do many things with the ashes; sprinkle them in their favourite place, create a space in gardens, and they also often hold onto them in the home. Lisa's ashes stayed in her wardrobe.

Tina and Colin said:

> *'People seemed to think we are strange, but where else would we keep them? She loved her clothes, she loved brightly coloured clothes, and she will be happy there in her wardrobe, in her bedroom.'*

However, keeping possessions can also create questions and issues, Tina, considering their potential house move in future, said:

> *'What will we do with her room and all her things? I can't get rid of anything, even scraps of paper which she has written on.'*

It was a parent at the mutual help group who helped her to find her answer.

> *'Before I moved her nail varnish, I painted each colour onto a card with its name – and I took photos of all the rooms . . . so I still have images of how things were, even though they've been changed.'*

These sections highlight how important it is that psychosocial support takes the client's perspective; these stories acknowledge how loss affects all aspects of life and that continuing relationships are often the essence of stories following a significant death (Klass, Silverman & Nickman, 1999).

New languages

Language of theories

Tina and Colin remembered that:

> *'We were given a book on stages and tasks through grief . . . Well, you read the books that say how it should be . . . that may be how it should be for one person but definitely not for us, we read it for interest sake, but . . .'*

Tina and Colin then saw a cognitive behavioural therapist; they were not sleeping and their GP had referred them specifically for this issue. This made them think about the was in which a counseller could best support them.

They reflected that:

> *'He had obviously never dealt with bereaved people before . . . nobody who had lost a child anyway . . . He said our lack of sleep was a problem, that therefore Lisa was a problem, problems are challenges that we needed to work through . . . I could feel myself getting really sort of wound up and I didn't want to go back, but I did want to tell him what I thought. I went back and said: "Lisa is not a problem, Lisa is dead; that is a fact – that's not a challenge . . . it's real. We've dealt with challenges, we have changed jobs, we've gone without money, we've done all that and those are challenges. Lisa's death you know that is fact."'*

When Tina explored this further she felt that the therapist had probably been using his own language, not thinking about their experience of the death of their child but relying on the language between professionals, that is, terminology and jargon.

'He's obviously used to dealing with different problems that could be dealt with if you look at it from a different viewpoint.' This wasn't appropriate in this situation, but it helped them to understand his reaction, and explain why in their view he could not cope with their story.

Language in community

About the mutual help group they attended, they explained:

> *'It's a social thing really, just to talk with other people who are normal like us (laughing), as opposed to talking to people who are normal like everybody else . . . it's nice to just socialise and have a laugh and talk about living.'*

> *'People say, "oh they are out and about, laughing and so on, and so they must be better sort of thing" – community of same experience understand – laughing and crying.'*

This quote also highlights the reality of the dual process model as identified by Stroebe and Schut (1999) that bereaved people move between grieving and diversion from grief quite naturally.

Tina notes her difficulties with describing her family:

> *'When somebody asks, "have you got children?" you think, how many do you say, or do you say two? It is your reaction and your feelings that are adjusted by their reactions. You don't want to block the conversation. It is a real conversation stopper isn't it really . . . I used to say "Anna's 22 and Lisa would have been 24" and I think that anybody who is sensitive would have picked up on it, and people who didn't weren't that interested anyway, so I used to get away with it like that.'*

And talking about Lisa in their real terms:

> *'We really needed to talk about Lisa as she was – she was fun, smiling, through all her disabilities, but she could also be difficult, very stubborn at times. People don't seem to want to hear that . . . I feel that they are thinking "she's dead, everything you say must be positive". I love her; it's just that at times I got tired and frustrated too.'*

Feelings: anger, guilt, sadness

Tina and Colin also discussed the impacts on their second child; feeling they were not doing enough for Lisa, they also both reflected that they believed they had neglected Anna both during Lisa's life and after her death.

'Lisa had been in intensive care for like 2 ½ weeks (she had been in and out of hospital for all of her short life) . . . It was six months before we found that she had actually died from the measles virus. We were so angry. Finally, she was on a ventilator, but there was a time when we knew she had had enough . . . so we decided to turn it off then.'

Having to make this decision caused them huge feelings of guilt, alongside sadness, as they had difficulty in accepting this decision and received no support through this time. In this interview they referred to the ensuing court case, but just mentioned that this was extremely stressful to them.

'We said we felt, sort of selfish . . . but she (the counsellor at specialist centre) turned it round - to "self full". Said we just had to, like, look after ourselves before everybody else and we realised if everybody else don't like it, tough. There was no right or wrong way. People may disagree but then we learnt it's probably their problem not ours.'

The power of emotions: 'walking around the rim of despair'

Tina described how she felt traumatised by her daughter's death; after seeing her dead on the bed with 'all the tubes removed', she started to have panic attacks. At this time Tina described herself like a 'rabbit caught in the lights', as she kept recalling and turning over the events. She was scared of talking about her emotions and fearful she would become depressed.

'It's sometimes like I'm walking around the rim, the edge of my despair, it's a huge abyss . . . I know where I am, and I can see the hole, a huge bottomless pit, and I don't know what's down the bottom, I'm scared if I go there . . . well I'll just never come out again.'

Tina's counsellor used this image to help her to understand her feelings; she helped her to explore how she was feeling at the time, to take a look into the pit and what it meant to her. The counsellor sensed, and let Tina know, that she felt she may need to take her time to really connect to her feelings of angst and grief and if she did she may need additional support around her, both from counselling, as well as from friends.

This couple demonstrate a difference in grief between men and women. In the first instance, Colin reacted to their daughter's death in a different way. He was more practical in his approach – 'What can we do, how shall we do it?' It was later that the full impact of his daughter's death really sank in and he expressed feelings of sadness, anger, guilt, and bitterness; his grief was really raw. The importance to them as a couple was that they went to sessions together; they could see how they were each reacting and responding to the situation and that this was different, but in the session they could explain this to each other, something they could not do at home. This highlights the frequent difference in the way we can grieve, how flexible we need to be in order to work with different 'ways of being' in the face of grief (Martin & Doka, 2000).

When does grief end?

Tina and Colin chose when to end their counselling – after 2 years. The following quote shows that they had no idea how long they would need to continue in counselling and even how off-putting it could have been for them if someone had told them at the outset that they could be there 2 years later:

> *'When we'd been there a few months, we wondered how long it takes; we heard somebody else saying it had been five years. It was a shock actually, and we thought we were nearly there then. It is completely open ended . . . we could go as long as we liked . . . the support was free but we chose to make donations.'*

However, this ability to choose an ending does not apply in all services, as illustrated below (expanding the quote used in Chapter 3).

Voices

Kirsten, a widow who received counselling from a national bereavement service, found her sessions were brought to a close when:

> *'. . . I'd only got to the crying stage, probably got onto the angry stage . . . because she said there are stages to grief . . . and that was when they cut it – they sliced it – and there was so much more that I was wanting to get out.'*

Kirsten

Kirsten continued to feel this way and subsequently contacted another bereavement service, who carried on her counselling until she made more adjustments to her life and began to feel more at ease about living without Steve.

This highlights how important it is that we make endings with clients at an appropriate time and in an appropriate manner. Arguably, an ending for a bereaved client who has faced a significant loss needs to be handled with additional care. Ending counselling sessions when a client has experienced a loss has also been identified as an area that raises considerable anxiety for counsellors (see Chapter 4).

Research has highlighted that in the best interests of the bereaved client the psychosocial service should be ongoing (Flatteau Taylor, 2003).

Summary

- Clients' whole lives are turned upside down by loss. Often these anxieties are feelings of immobilisation – shock and trauma – like a rabbit in the headlights, as is often reported in the early days of grief. Clients need proactive guidance to access counselling; they need someone to provide some understanding, to find the right place, the right service, at the right time.
- Clients also need:
  - Services to be sensitive to, and flexible about, the setting of their counselling (without presumption of what is right).
  - To talk about everything – after the initial splash of that rock in the pool, the ripple effect of loss affects all aspects of life.
  - Services which will 'go the distance' and stay alongside bereaved people for as long as it takes, as grief is not resolved, and has no ending.
  - Counsellors to understand that they do not fit grief into patterns or theories – grief is about all of life; there are no stages or tasks.
- These client's stories also ask counsellors to:
  - Let me be with my relationship with the deceased – don't make me feel mad because I feel her inside me, hear her voice.
  - Don't go ahead of me and show me what is there.
  - Don't go behind me – or take me to the past until I am ready, if I am ready to go there.
  - Just be alongside me – I need to talk about everything – I need my own timescale.

    - Accept me; help me to accept myself and to explore how I am coping.
    - Be honest with me.
- It is about 'being' not 'doing'.
- I use the quote at the start of this chapter to remind myself constantly of the privileged place I am in when clients talk about their whole lives to me, and to respect what they need to talk about, and how scary it can be to talk about all aspects of life.

The specialist service that Tina and Colin eventually found, provided this for them, and they said 'If we hadn't found that centre . . . God knows where we would be now.'

Activity

Think of a loss that you have experienced in your own life; how do your experiences link in with the clients' voices in this chapter?

Further reading

I would suggest here a mix of literature; hearing clients' voices is extremely important so to read about direct experience as well as fiction can be useful, but also look at different aspects of grief.

Laird, E. (1988) *Red Sky in the Morning*. Oxford: Heinemann.

Lewis, C. S. (2001) *A Grief Observed*. London: HarperOne.

Martin, T. and Doka, K. (2000) *Men Don't Cry, Women Do: Transcending Gender Stereotypes of Grief*. Philadelphia PA: Brunner Mazel.

Chapter 7
Professional challenges

'What does Crustimoney Proseedcake mean?' said Pooh (. . .) 'It means the Thing to Do.' Said Owl

A. A. Milne

Traditionally the 'professions' comprised doctors, engineers, lawyers, architects and commissioned military officers. These were people who undertook a specialised set of tasks for a fee. Today the adjective 'professional' is applied more broadly to paid and voluntary roles and relates to the provision of a good quality of service.

This is quite a formal chapter, which takes a look at some influences on our role as professionals in the specialist field of loss and bereavement. While we are doing this, let's not forget to have a smile as well, as we translate our own 'customary procedures' and turn them around, think of them differently – perhaps a little like Pooh bear as in the quote above!

This chapter will include:

- Employment
  - Role, job title, job specification
  - Specialism and expertise
  - Career opportunities
  - Working in a team and managing a team
- Referral pathways and information
  - Raising awareness about the service
  - Referral pathways
- Quality control, evaluation and monitoring the impacts of our work
  - Training of counsellors
  - Evaluation and monitoring
  - Supervision
  - Complaints, grievance and 'whistle-blowing'
- Research
- Finance and funding
- Summary

Let's take a look at what effects working with loss may have within a practice. Whether we are working as single practitioners, or as managers, the focus and standard of our work may be affected by the following aspects.

Employment

Role, job title and job specification

It is important to ensure that we are working within the parameters of our role, our training and qualification. We need to be able to understand our job title, job description or person specification in order not simply to provide a framework for our practice, but also to explain our role to our clients.

Even the job title can and will impact on our 'professional pride', as illustrated in the following example.

Change in job title

A staff member at the Maypole Project was employed as a 'family support assistant' student counsellor to denote that she was not yet qualified to diploma level. On gaining her counselling diploma, she was offered a new title of 'family support practitioner', reflecting her newly qualified status. She was delighted. This change helped her to define herself professionally within the service, with clients, and colleagues in other services.

Note: Since plans for registration were scrapped by the current government (December 2012) the BACP is now piloting a Certificate of Proficiency scheme as a second tier for counsellors who do not meet the requirements for accreditation. This involves taking a test to prove ability, which would allow them to be approved to practice but not be accredited. More information is available on the BACP website.

As counsellors we frequently define our role through our theoretical stance or professional qualification such as 'art therapist' or 'cognitive behavioural therapist'; our role may be defined by our client group as in 'relationship or family therapist', or through the specialist issues we may work with such as 'addiction', 'loss' and 'bereavement'.

In the context of working with loss, the title of 'bereavement counsellor' or 'counsellor who works in loss and bereavement' will have an impact on us. A brief reference in Chapter 1 starts a discussion about how the first may denote a counsellor who is more focused on working with the loss in his or her clients' life, while the second may reflect a more holistic approach. We also need to be aware that in addition to impacting on our professional pride, our job title may be an indicator as to how we intend to provide counselling to people facing bereavement.

Services differ greatly in the counselling they offer people facing loss. As counsellors, we need to be sure that we are aware of the ethos and working practices of our service, and that the role we apply for and take on has a good enough 'fit' with our way of working; it is important not to compromise integrity with the need for a job. It is quite unlikely that the service will change or adapt to our way of working, but whether they will incorporate our differences may be an important question to reflect on during interview.

Specialism and expertise

So we have chosen our pathway, secured a post as a counsellor and if that role is clearly specialist, the inference is that we would be trained in a particular area of a subject. Of course, this could apply to any counsellor but may not be incorporated within their job title but what if our name does depict us as specialists, what does this mean to us professionally, to our colleagues and, most importantly, to our clients?

If we are portrayed as 'the experts', this could have differing effects. Clients may see us as proficient and skillful and able to provide them with the answers to their questions. If they ask questions such as, 'When will grief end?', how do we respond?

Professional recognition of such expertise may lead to other professionals deferring to our expertise, which may 'tap into' our ego and image of self. Similarly, it could raise anxieties, with such high expectations placed upon us.

Loss and bereavement is sometimes referred to as a 'niche' by counselling professionals. This could imply that 'yes we are experts... but only in loss and bereavement'. In other words, a specialism can refer to just bereavement. The assumption here is that as we work 'on the edge' of counselling, with a specific set of issues, we may not have knowledge or experience in other areas. Others may believe that with specialist training we could become more employable in a specialist loss setting, and less employable in a more generic service.

My personal experience has been of generalist training with placements in loss and bereavement, followed by an ongoing career in loss and bereavement alongside which I run a private practice. I have been employed to work in a children's behaviour support team and counselled people with a range of presenting issues. The holistic way I practice, in whichever setting, means I have worked with many issues including: different deaths, terminations, and other aspects of loss including divorce, sexual, physical and emotional abuse, addiction, eating disorders, long-term chronic illnesses, adoption, fostering and people presenting with low mood or chronic anxiety. Yet I still remain known as a specialist in loss and bereavement. So what really is a specialism?

My belief is that if you are trained to deal with loss you will be able to work in most areas as loss is linked to just about every presenting issue.

A specialist role implies specialist training, and posts for counsellors working in loss frequently request that applicants have 'at least 2 years' post-qualifying experience in working in loss'. How does this work in practice?

In a recent recruitment drive for a family support practitioner, the initial role outline and person specification highlighted the need for a minimum of two years' experience in loss and bereavement as noted. The rationale for this was to gain interest and applications from counsellors for whom loss had some resonance. We employed a therapist who had not in fact worked in a specialist role but who could demonstrate an ability to work and empathise with bereaved clients. In the interview we also asked 'Why this organisation?', 'Why this role?' and 'Why now?'.

Career opportunities

There are many career opportunities for those working in loss: from the more obvious bereavement services and hospice services to counselling services within hospitals. These services and titles sometimes belie the fact that they are providing support following a loss, for example The

Maypole Project or Women's Health Counsellor (in a hospital setting). The different settings in which counsellors work with loss are outlined in Chapter 2, which may provide some ideas about potential career opportunities. But think about the different losses which are outlined in the introduction and the different types of death outlined in Chapter 4. The ongoing message of this book is that loss is all around us. Within the voluntary sector there are many charities that work with people, dealing with specific non-death related losses.

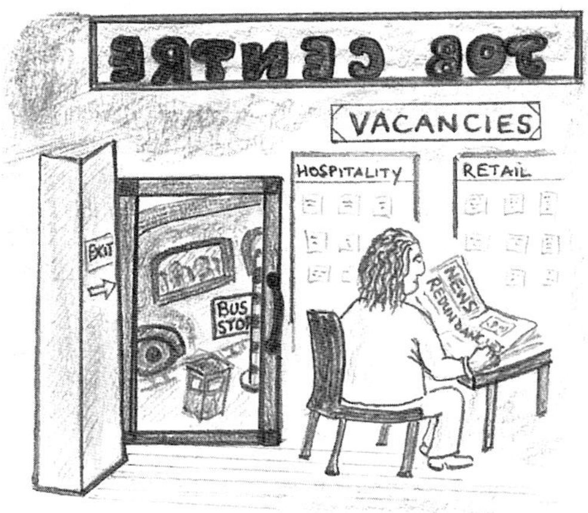

Figure 7.1 Career opportunities

Working in a team/managing a team

Team work can bring additional tensions for counsellors, particularly in the areas of communication, confidentiality and at times dual roles. At the Maypole Project the families are explicitly offered confidentiality 'within the organisation'. This is explained at our initial meeting with families in the following terms.

Confidentiality

'Sarah will be your family support practitioner – your main point of contact. However, in this small organisation the whole team is involved with all aspects of the service, and they will (on a need-to-know basis) know your family name, but they will have no details of your personal/private issues discussed in support.'

Alison, a parent accessing counselling, reflected that this is a bit like 'being one of the Maypole family'. She said, 'I really appreciate being known and knowing some staff; it means I can phone and leave messages easily.' She has also noted her appreciation of the limitations on staff knowledge of her full story.

The Maypole Project offers support to all family members, which may include counselling, befriending and activities for children. From these services the families can individually and/or collectively create their own holistic package of psychosocial care. This can sometimes lead to a counsellor having dual relationships with the family. The BACP Ethical Framework (2010) notes that dual relationships may have:

> 'a powerful beneficial or detrimental impact that may not always be easily foreseeable'.
>
> **BACP Ethical Framework (2010)**

In order to overcome any adverse effects, it is essential that the members of staff concerned have a discussion to highlight any possibilities of conflicts/detrimental effects for their client(s) and work out ways to avoid this situation, should it arise. It is also important to note that all eventualities may not be identified immediately so this consideration needs to be ongoing. Dialogues should also be held with the client, who needs to be aware of the possibility that he or she may meet their counsellor in another role, or in different situations and to consider what impact this may have, and how or whether they wish their relationship to be acknowledged.

The tension of managing a multidisciplinary team is that this openness is balanced with a 'need to know'; for example, that conversations about clients are never held across an open office and do not breach confidentiality. While working in a team brings many issues, like those mentioned above, it also lessens counsellors' experience of isolation and provides more opportunities to discuss areas of concern.

A further tension can lie in a dual role of line management and supervision. When this occurs the initial impact can be foreseen, but ongoing discussion and exploration is needed in order to ensure that relationships and the work are running easily for both parties.

Referral pathways and information

Raising awareness about the service

All services – whether single practices or larger services – need to consider publicity. Materials may be produced in the form of leaflets or posters and distributed around the community, or at points from which clients may be referred such as doctors' surgeries; or advertisements may be placed in the press or counselling journals. We must ensure that the message we portray about our counselling is honest and representative; and that nothing is suggested or stated which may be deemed to be unprofessional, detrimental to clients or misleading. In loss and bereavement, this will relate to the way in which we state we work with loss and represent the 'grieving process'.

Referral pathways

Managers have the responsibility to ensure that counsellors fully understand all aspects of the service provision including referral pathways and referral criteria, in order that they can discuss this accurately with clients. Effective communication through the service is essential, although it is important to know that this can at times raise issues surrounding confidentiality.

Quality control, evaluation and monitoring the impacts of our work

Control of quality in counselling can be monitored in several ways including effective selection and recruitment as outlined above, through training, evaluation and monitoring, finding a supervisor, and effective policies such as those referring to complaints, grievance and whistle-blowing.

Training of counsellors

A trawl of generic counselling courses shows that the majority include loss and bereavement in their curriculum. However, from speaking to peers in researching this book, from clients' stories, and from counsellors I have worked with, the content is quite limited, giving scope for further in-depth training. This is echoed in Chapter 4, which highlights the many anxieties raised due to lack of background knowledge. It is also important that we continually update our knowledge, current theories and thinking around bereavement and provide space for personal reflection on the subject. Many courses incorporate the theories of stages, phases, tasks and exclude the more contemporary theoretical developments. Chapter 5 notes the importance of effective training; here we need to look at its significance to us, and identify any courses we need.

It is easy to become slightly confused when attempting to understand bereavement qualifications; there are courses available entitled 'Diploma in Bereavement Counselling', which will provide insight and teaching around issues of loss and bereavement, together with counselling skills, but there are none, to my knowledge, which would fulfill sufficient training in counselling to be considered to be at counselling diploma level. However, for those who already have a counselling diploma, such courses may provide additional continual professional development training to expand their knowledge sufficiently to apply for a counselling post in loss and bereavement. Some specialist training programmes are detailed in Chapter 10, and you will see that these are frequently connected to specialist services, so it would be useful to contact your local hospice or bereavement service for further information. The level of this training and its content are not currently regulated.

From the perspective of counselling students, the experience gained in a placement within bereavement has often been insufficient for the requirements of the course; tutors request students to take additional placements that are not 'just bereavement'. This would demonstrate that tutors see bereavement as a specialist subject which is limited and limiting for the student.

Evaluation and monitoring

As counsellors, we may not necessarily become involved in the evaluation of our support; however, it is important to include it here, as it is an area which informs our level of professional performance.

Knowing a little about the client's perspective is an essential piece of information for counsellors. I often hear of counsellors who work in loss and bereavement struggling when working with clients who have faced a major loss in life. The counselling comes to a close, and sometimes there is no greatly noticeable difference. Where possible, it is extremely helpful to gain the client's perspective on his or her counselling experience.

Supervision

In order to maintain our professional standards as counsellors, we need to access supervision to the level that is prescribed by our membership, or accrediting body. But what effect, if any, does working in loss and bereavement have on finding a supervisor? In addition to the usual role of supervision, when we are working in loss and bereavement our supervisor needs to be able to support us in working in an intense, sometimes traumatic and always sensitive area. From a supervisor, we need additional educational input which facilitates the integration and understanding of the client's experiences with the theories of loss and grief.

Through supervision we should also be encouraged to deepen our self-awareness, understand process issues at an interpersonal and intrapersonal level and reflect on transference and counter-transference as it arises in the bereavement work with clients. To my knowledge, there is no register of supervisors who specialise in loss and bereavement. For me, finding a supervisor with suitable qualifications and experience whom I could also relate to on a personal level has been a case of trial and error. Across the years, I found a supervisor who provided the high support I needed at the start, but I quickly reached a point where I needed more learning and challenge. I moved to a supervisor who again provided high support, but the challenge here arose when I noted that her approach differed from mine and my placements; this transpired to be because she was working from her own experience of loss and needs at that time. It took five years to meet Jim Kuykendall, the supervisor who has provided the ideal balance: helping me to integrate my humanistic counselling with a deep understanding of the existential angst of clients facing loss and bereavement.
We quickly developed a robust relationship that was both supportive and challenging.

Voices

On starting with the service, a counsellor became anxious about a client, and said in supervision:

> *'My client is talking about her son's behaviour, not about her mum who's died. I feel she is deflecting from talking about her death. Should I let her talk, should we refer her on . . . is she in the right place?'*

Counsellor

Let's unpack this and reflect. With the statement, 'My client is talking about her son' a subject is raised that does not in itself 'fit' the criteria for referral; that is, death. The supervisor encouraged the counsellor to explore the sessions more and asked whether she felt that the client connected this behaviour to her mum's death. The answer was 'yes'; the behaviour resulted from years of caring for her mum at home, their relationship had become strained and her son had felt neglected. In this service setting, this was clearly then within the remit of this counsellor's role.

Complaints, grievances and 'whistle-blowing'

Instances of complaints, grievances and 'whistle-blowing' can be followed on a month-by-month basis through the sanction pages in the BACP Therapy Today. We must be aware that as counsellors we have the obligation not only to make appropriate space and process that will allow our clients to make complaints. It is also our duty to bring to the attention of the appropriate bodies any issues of bad practice we may see. Services should have due process for dealing with these issues.

Research

Keeping updated with current research is crucial to ensure we demonstrate a duty of care and quality control for our clients. However, we may also engage in research. The challenges facing counsellors who feel anxious about accessing, contributing to, or conducting research are outlined in Challenges for Counsellors: Research, by Jim Carmichael (2013). Additionally, there are issues surrounding the sensitivity of the subject of loss and bereavement. If as counsellors we engage in qualitative studies through interviews/ethnography, we should ensure that we do not unduly disturb our clients, and offer additional independent support for them subsequent to the interview. It was interesting to note that one outcome of 'Between the idea and the Reality' (Flatteau Taylor, 2005) was that on being offered additional support post-interview, 80 per cent of participants stated they felt that the interview process had helped them in their grief rather than created difficulties. Another challenge noted was holding the tension of being a researcher: providing interviews, rather than providing a counselling session.

Finance and funding

A core challenge for services can be concerns regarding funding. Counselling services often enter into contracts with other providers to provide specialist counselling, which can result in the counselling being provided free of charge to the user. In a voluntary/charity setting there tend to be several funding streams, but fundraising is often the main route. It is important that the organisation offering a free service does not place an underlying, unspoken pressure on clients to either make a donation, or fundraise for them. Managers should note other potential underlying pressures; firstly that clients may feel that they should minimise their uptake of sessions because they are not paying for them. Secondly, they should also be aware of potential pressure on counsellors to limit the service they provide.

Guidelines, policies and procedures

A Department of Health report notes that many bereavement services within the NHS have evolved as a result of local 'champions', with a particular interest in bereavement. This has resulted in provision which tends to be reactive rather than proactive, with a notable lack of standardised guidelines, policies and procedures related to information, monitoring uptake, follow up, and onward referral (DH, 2012). It is important then that specific policies relating to loss and bereavement are in place; for example, what to do if:

- counsellors face a loss in their lives
- the team need support through a critical incident including debrief, and additional one-to-one support.

Summary

- While we want to avoid blurring the boundaries, it is important that we do not split our professional issues in a way in which we disown our personal issues. We should remember that what affects us professionally will also affect us to a greater or lesser degree personally. It is also important to bear in mind that any professional issues we may have could be evident to, or affect, our clients.
- It is of vital importance that we remain professional when working with loss; we will be working with sensitive issues that require us to be able to simply 'be' with our client. This is an impossible task if we have various professional anxieties racing through our minds.
- It is also important that we update our specialist knowledge and look for jobs that fit our methods of working, so that we can support our clients to the absolute best of our ability.

Activity

Read about the issues presented in this chapter around job titles for counselling for those working in loss.

Do they capture issues you may have considered?

What would you add to this discussion, or change?

How do you think that job title may affect someone looking for counselling following a loss?

Further reading

Information about standards and guidelines for loss and bereavement and training courses/centres can be found in the appendix.

Chapter 8

Ethical challenges

'Compassion, in which all ethics must take root . . .'

Albert Schweitzer

As counsellors, our first aim is the duty of care to our clients. To this end it is imperative that we create an environment and trusting relationship within which clients feel able to explore their issues, and talk about the most intimate and sensitive areas of their lives. To do this, we need to be able to demonstrate our ability to be compassionate, professional and ethical in our work.

While recognising the many ethical guidelines available, for ease of reference this chapter takes the BACP Ethical Framework as a structure, highlighting any impacts of working with clients who are facing loss and bereavement, alongside its key themes. This will cover the effects of loss and bereavement on the framework we create, in addition to the impact from 'inside' the relationship, how we may be affected by issues presented by our clients that contain their values and beliefs, which may differ greatly from our own. These guidelines cannot provide a comprehensive, fully inclusive set of rules for our work; however, they present us with underpinning ethical and moral values by which we should work.

This chapter will include:

- What are ethics: why do we need them?
- What are ethics as applied to counselling?
  - Honour the trust placed in us (fidelity)
  - Respect the client's right to be self-directing (autonomy)
  - Promote the client's well being (beneficence)
  - Do no harm (maleficence) – *premum non nocere* (Latin)

What are ethics: why do we need them?

Ethics centre on a concern about something, or someone, other than ourselves and our own desires and self-interest. Ethical guidelines can therefore provide a 'moral map' as a system of honourable principles, affecting how people lead their lives and make decisions. They are concerned with what is good for society and individuals.

As ethics are not necessarily 'absolute truths', they provide guidelines rather than rules: a backbone from which we can construct our counselling practice. They can instruct us when our heart or 'gut instinct' may be at odds with our knowledge or 'head'. Our moral obligation encompassed in such guidelines is to aspire to the personal qualities of: empathy, sincerity, integrity, resilience, respect, humility, competence, fairness, wisdom, and courage (BACP, 2010).

This then is the foundation of the safety of our work.

The provision of ethical services starts from the basic principals of: clarity and appropriateness of information about service, content of initial meetings, and the parameters within which we provide counselling (BACP, 2010). This outline is a means by which counsellors can be 'policed': the starting point to ensure the safety and measure the quality of counselling. Ethical guidelines will need to cover all aspects of counselling, from our capability to carry out our role to our personal well being, through to the level of training and supervision we receive.

The basic tenets of ethics are outlined below and, where appropriate, there is specific reference to issues faced when working with clients who are bereaved. As counsellors, when facing our clients it will be impossible to choose and apply appropriate principles as a generality; we need to use our insight, with additional input from our supervisors and line managers, as each case will be uniquely different. However, as counsellors our obligation is:

> to consider all the relevant circumstances with as much care as is reasonably possible and to be appropriately accountable for decisions made.
>
> BACP, 2010

What are ethics as applied to counselling?

An essential start point of any counselling must be the formation of a relationship in which mutual trust is established.

Being trustworthy: honouring the trust placed in us

I am constantly amazed by clients who, even at a first session, will open the most intimate areas of their life to me. But it is vital to remember that even though we are there to listen, it is not our automatic right to be trusted. Firstly, we need to be demonstrably trustworthy.

Achieving this can start even before counselling begins through clarity of information about the service. Then when we first meet with clients we can contract with them. Stop there! Will I be seen as trustworthy if I use language which confuses? What a 'contract' means may be clear to us but often is not clear to clients. We have already touched on the barrier that jargon and terminology can create in the counselling relationship.

Contracting is about providing information about the service, our role with the client, any limitations to the service. In providing counselling for loss and bereavement, this may also include specific information about the counselling to be provided; whether the sessions will be totally focused on the client's experience of death and bereavement, or whether a more holistic approach may be taken. This needs to be clear in order that the client can make an informed choice about whether this is the appropriate service for them.

It is essential that this information is totally understood and carefully integrated into our work, so that what we do matches what we say we will do. The foundation of such information will be held in the detail of policies held by the service such as:

- mission statement: outlining the service's values and aims, its referral criteria
- who the service is supporting, when, where, the parameters of the service
- length of service: brief intervention, long term
- the way of working: cognitive behavioural therapy, person centred.

Policies also need to focus on ourselves as counsellors and include issues of health and safety and working alone in different settings, monitoring our levels of competence and ability to work.

Policies and procedures are vital in creating a trustworthy environment. Where they are thoroughly embedded in the service and integrated into the working pattern, they will ensure that services are appropriate and safe, delivered appropriately to clients. Such policies also ensure our safety and well being in the delivery of counselling.

First and foremost clients note that the privacy of a service and its promise of confidentiality is an essential base. This will reflect respect for our clients and their stories, with the limitations outlined in the BACP guidelines for confidentiality. Loss and bereavement is a sensitive subject and some aspects or types of loss encompass additional sensitivities. It is important that when offering counselling we are aware of any potential additional need for confidentiality, as shown in the following example.

Anna

Anna was referred to a specialist bereavement service following the death of a family friend. Having gained trust in her counsellor, she revealed that this family friend had been her lover for 10 years. Her family and other friends knew she was grieving his loss, but did not know this full story, so she hid the depth and intensity of her grief from others.

This case raised some questions for the counsellor. Anna was certain that people would think her strange to request counselling for the death of a friend (although this is a frequent reason for referral). Absolute care had to be taken to ensure that no trace of the referral was made public; no letters were to be sent and no telephone messages were to be left, even on her mobile phone. During this work the counsellor identified some personal moral difficulties, a level of disapproval regarding her client's bereavement from the death of a lover, which she took to supervision. This she subsequently discussed within her personal therapy to ensure that she supported her client without clouding from her own values and beliefs.

A further example of ethics 'in action' has arisen during the writing of this book. I participated in a Radio 4 programme Inside the Ethics Committee, which focused on the treatment (through tracheostomy) of two children who had degenerative diseases. My initial reservations were strong: I did not have the experience of medical ethics and I would not in my practice come to conclusions or make decisions about treatment. However, as a persuasive researcher explained that the aim of the role was to provide expert insight into the reactions and needs of the children and families, I realised that every day I sit alongside clients who make such hugely difficult decisions. In addition, working with clients who discuss such issues brings up issues for me, and I need to check that I am in no way steering them, but stay alongside them in their decisions/reactions to situations.

This ties in with the next section. We need to respect the client's ability and right to be self-governing; this starts from the information we provide about the service, and how clients access the service.

Autonomy: respect for the client's right to be self-governing

As counsellors, we need to focus on the non-manipulation of clients and respect them in developing their ability to direct their own therapy and, indeed, way of life. In advance of services being offered and commencing, we need to provide clear information about the services we provide through promotions, advertising and referring organisations.

Informed consent is an essential aspect of the confidential and private service we provide. The BACP guidelines state:

> 'All routine referrals to colleagues and other services should be discussed with the client in advance and the client's consent obtained both to making the referral and also to disclosing information to accompany the referral.'
>
> BACP, 2010

However, note some potential tensions here between guideline and practice.

Referrals by GPs

A bereavement service created a referral route from general practitioners across one borough. The outline above (BACP, 2010) was the guideline for referrals. However, GPs chose the following routes for their patients who had faced a death, which were:

- referral on request of counselling
- information provision to bereaved patients so they could self-refer
- 'blanket' referral of all bereaved patients, with information in the surgery about the link to the bereavement service.

On evaluation the highest level of satisfaction with the timing and process of referral was through self-referral and 'blanket' referral (Flatteau Taylor, 2003).

As bereaved people feel as though they are in 'no man's land' after a death, they report needing a more proactive approach in helping them to access counselling.

It is vital that we bring any conflicts of interest to our clients' awareness as soon as possible. Here is an example of how this responsibility starts within us. In loss and bereavement, our conflicts of interest may relate to our ability to work with clients presenting with different aspects of loss. Training needs to ensure that we explore any areas of loss, which we feel we may be less able to work with and this, in turn, should be monitored through supervision. Conflict may arise through a duality of roles with the client. Whether these are previously known or emerge, such as a chance meeting in a different place, the client's confidentiality and right to privacy should be respected and made freely available at all times.

Beneficence: a commitment to promoting the client's well being

The most important element in this commitment is ensuring that we are working to the limits of our ability and competence. It is key when working with loss and bereavement to gain an understanding of the impacts of loss on people, on society and most importantly on the practitioner. This should then be monitored through supervision/ training and continuing professional development (CPD). It is essential that a supervisor has either specialist knowledge in loss and bereavement, or access to additional information/support from a specialist, in order to monitor both ability and current competence. Training and updating practice through CPD enhances the quality of our work. Issues pertaining to training courses are explored further in Chapter 7.

A continual review of our knowledge base and an integration of updated research into our practice are essential in ensuring that we provide the best possible counselling to our clients. Mary, in the example below, felt that her counsellor was working to a framework of stage theories that did not fit her experience; however, Chapter 3 highlights how new theories are emerging which provide an insight into the bereavement process as a more fluid and dynamic experience.

Voices

Mary felt her counsellor put some pressure on her, wanting her to demonstrate her grief, to highlight her stage of grief. She said

> *'I think she wanted something that I wasn't giving her, I felt that . . . If I started to cry I stopped myself and I think she would have preferred it if I let rip, but I couldn't. The counsellor said that I have got stuck in the bereavement process, I haven't moved on . . . through different stages . . . I haven't felt it in actual stages as such – just desolation. Complete and utter desolation . . . awfulness.'*

Mary in Flatteau Taylor, 2005

BACP Ethical Guidelines (2010) stress the importance of the inclusion of clients whose capacity for autonomy may be diminished due to circumstances such as extreme distress or serious disturbance. This is highly applicable to clients who are facing loss, as they may be suffering a complete emotional upheaval and shock. These guidelines advocate that when clients are seriously disturbed, information needs to be provided clearly, carefully and repeated regularly, with time allowed to check for understanding. This will help to ensure that the client is really able to process any implications of the information provided. This must also be applied where a client is more immature, or lacking in understanding due to learning disabilities, or has a different first language, or is from a different culture. It is important that ease of access to information is created for all clients.

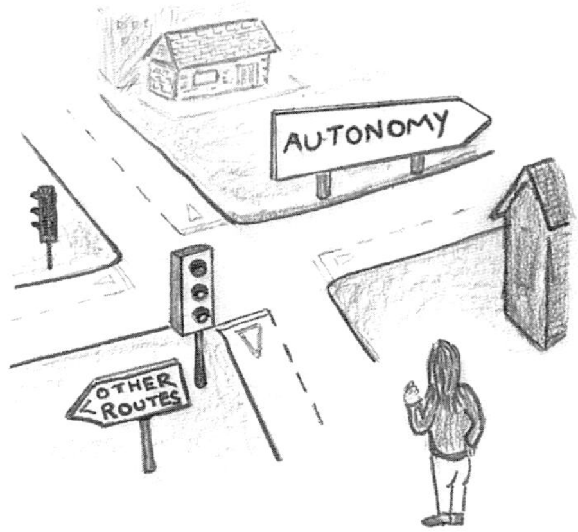

Figure 8.1 Autonomy

Non-maleficence: a commitment to avoiding harm to the client

This involves avoiding any form of exploitation of clients; this may be sexual, financial or emotional, or from harmful methods of practice such as incompetence or malpractice. This may be apparent and overt, but such exploitation can also be subtle and covert. A respondent to research outlined her experience of a counselling relationship which became abusive.

Voices

'After about six months of counselling, I'd told him a lot about me, about deaths I'd experienced as rejections, about people controlling me and my life. . . then in a way after a while I became his counsellor, he was telling me everything about his personal life . . . I always felt like he controlled me.'

Helen in Flatteau Taylor, 2005

This vignette demonstrates the beginnings of the clear allegations by the respondent that her counsellor was breaking boundaries. As an interviewer,

I took these issues to my supervisor to seek information about the need to address her allegations of malpractice by this counsellor. However, having talked through the experience in this interview my supervisor informed me that she had begun to take a complaint forward with support from another counsellor, so my input was not needed.

To avoid harm to the client we also need to be able to monitor our level of ability or inability to work through personal circumstances. For example, as counsellors working with loss we may face the issue of loss in our own lives. Here's my personal experience.

> When my dad became ill many years ago several things happened: on one level I knew I needed to take time out to visit him in hospital. I wanted to be near him. At the same time, I was also conscious that I needed to ensure that my clients would be safe enough. Some days I knew I could function well, while on other days my mind and certainly my heart were not with my clients. The most important aspect for me was being aware that there was a policy in place that I could refer to and 'permit myself' time out. This policy outlines self-responsibility and self-regulation through accessing additional support. I added in extra supervision hours and therapy through this time to help me to monitor my professional ability and I also ensured I had others who would support me personally.

Justice: the fair and impartial treatment of all clients and the provision of adequate services

In principle, justice requires us to respect the human rights and dignity of our clients, staying alert to potential conflicts between legal and ethical tensions and/or obligations. Justice in distribution of services means that we must provide equal opportunities, appreciate diversity and difference, avoid discrimination and ensure equal distribution and allocation of services between clients. An example of difficulties in this area within a bereavement service is given below.

A GP referral noted 'Urgent Referral'

The client had been bereaved by suicide, and the GP added:

> *'this patient is extremely distraught and needs to talk to someone as soon as possible, preferably within a week'.*

This highlights the need for a responsive service but one that treats each case individually and, while acknowledging that a referrer may perceive that a client should be seen urgently, the service needs to stop and consider its caseload/waiting list, and also explore whether this could be the need of the referrer rather than of the prospective client.

Self-respect

The principle of self-respect means that the practitioner appropriately applies all the above values as entitlements for self-care. This includes seeking personal counselling and other opportunities for personal development as required. There is an ethical responsibility to use supervision for appropriate personal and professional support and development and to seek training and other opportunities for continuing professional development.

The principle of self-respect also encourages active engagement in life-enhancing activities and relationships that are independent of relationships in counselling or psychotherapy; exercises to help us identify such activities are illustrated in Chapter 5.

Alongside ensuring that professional standards are maintained in the work we carry out, counsellors also need to protect themselves against potential financial liabilities arising from complaints, as, soberingly, many complaints that have resulted in BACP sanctions can be seen in Therapy Today and these can quickly escalate into court cases. Insurance will give us a 'safety net', which hopefully we will not need to use, but such an assurance that should we need the backing of the law, both the service and the individual will be financially protected is very helpful in alleviating stress.

Summary

- The challenges and diversities in counselling mean that practitioners will inevitably encounter situations in which there are competing obligations.
- Our first duty to clients is 'premum non nocere', first do no harm. Bereaved people have already faced the most devastating of life's experiences, and it is essential that the counselling we provide alleviates rather than exacerbates the issues they face.
- Counselling people facing loss and bereavement raises some additional ethical issues, both of the framework in which we provide counselling and of the content of counselling itself.
- While a statement of ethics cannot take away difficulties in making professional judgements, such information can be of great assistance by providing guidelines that may need to be taken into consideration.

Activity

How do the issues above reflect the service you are working in?

Are there additional issues which you feel could be added for consideration?

Are there areas you had not considered?

Further reading

British Association for Counselling and Psychotherapy (BACP) (2010) Ethical Framework for Good Practice in Counselling & Psychotherapy.

Counselling and Psychotherapy in Scotland (COSCA) (2007) Statement of Ethics and Code of Practice.

British Psychological Society (2008) General Professional Practice Guidelines (2nd edn) Professional Practice Board.

Chapter 9
Research

'Between the idea and the reality, between the motion and the act falls the shadow.'

T. S. Eliot

The importance of informing our counselling practice through the integration of up-to-date ideas and research has been highlighted throughout this book and is further explored in the first two sections of this chapter. A paper by Jordan suggests that:

> ***'Most grief counsellors can articulate the models of mourning and recovery that guide their care giving . . . rather than the findings of research.'***
>
> Jordan, 2000: 461

The third section of this chapter outlines some of the few studies which explore the 'inside' of the counselling relationship with bereaved clients, in order to explore Jordan's view further. In the final section, just a few of the studies available on different aspects of loss and bereavement are outlined, illustrating the breadth of the subject, and linking to journals for further study (details are contained in the additional information given in the appendix).

This chapter will include:

- The importance of research
  - Who is involved?
- How do we find it? Why do we need it?
- When the two worlds of research and counselling practice meet
- Learning from our clients
- Specific areas of loss: the diversity of death in research
- Summary

The importance of research

Research is the study of materials and sources in order to establish facts and reach new conclusions, which may then become theories and accepted models. The word 'research' stems from the French, 'chercher', which in simple terms means 'to look for', or 'rechercher' which means to 'to look for again'. Rechercher provides the best 'fit' with this chapter, as here I will focus on 'looking again' for research, identifying studies that investigate what is happening 'in action' within counselling, which theories and models are being used, and whether they can outline different ways of working.

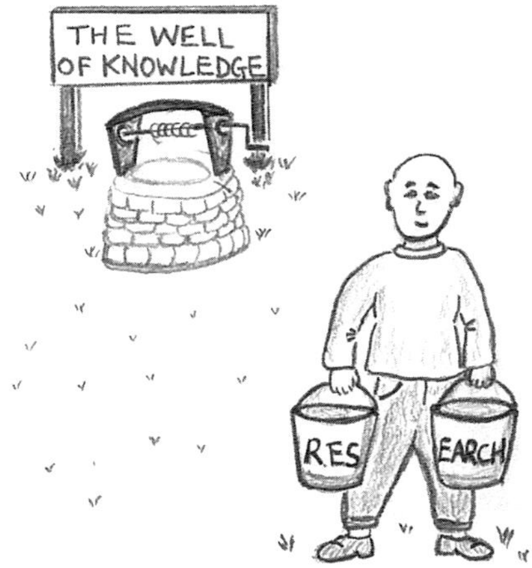

Figure 9.1 Chercher and Rechercher – The well of knowledge

Who is involved?

Quite simply all counsellors are involved, whether we are research practitioners or simply aim to keep up to date with our knowledge of subjects to integrate into practice. This chapter aims to provide an outline of several examples of updated research and to consider the ease of access to updated research and resources for continued study.

How do we find it, why do we need it?

The answer to these questions in my experience has come from both training and supervision. Training is our first 'port of call' for information and learning about counselling, and supervision is our ongoing source of input when we start out in placements and practice.

My first counselling placement, co-facilitating a widows support group, demonstrated to me the breadth of people's experiences on bereavement and, alongside this, the supervisor directed me to additional reading. Both of these experiences ran parallel to my personal experience of the death of five close family members within the previous couple of years, but jarred with the idea of stages and tasks that I had been taught. This discord prompted me to search further into this area, resulting in the outline of studies given briefly below. While different courses will have many differing approaches, I have found the theoretical base of stages and tasks in bereavement to be the centre of study for the many counsellors and counselling students I now supervise. A study of psychology textbooks also found that Kübler-Ross's stage theory (1971) was well presented, but other theoretical views were largely absent (Coppola and Strohmetz, 2002).

There are many books written around loss and bereavement and there are several professional and research journals that focus on death, loss and bereavement, some of which are listed in the appendix. It is worth making an internet search for specific papers, but be aware that without a subscription or having university access to publications, these usually need to be purchased.

The following sections provide the client's view on what works best for them, as well as highlighting how counsellors, counselling education and literature appear to have become 'hooked' on theories that some researchers view as out-dated. We'll identify access to more current research and introduce new ways of thinking, which we can integrate into our counselling practice.

When the two worlds of research and counselling practice meet

This section will outline some studies that explore the potential for a 'gap' between research and practice in thanatology (Jordan, 2000). Jordan somewhat powerfully suggests that:

> '. . . there is convincing evidence that many of the clinical constructs that have guided bereavement interventions over the years may not be much more than collectively shared assumptions . . . intervention research could add much to our knowledge about what will actually work in the "real" and uncontrolled settings where most caregivers operate.'
>
> **Jordan, 2000: 461**

The studies outlined here will provide insight into the counselling work itself, primarily from the client's perspective, to see which models have been integrated into counselling practices and aim to identify what works. Bereaved people continue to seek counselling following a loss, so it is vital that we try to get it right when providing them with support. I will outline in more detail some studies which relate the client's story directly, in order to ascertain what bereaved people need.

Learning from our clients

When research into counselling from the bereaved client's perspective has been carried out (and such studies are scarce), the focus is often on outcomes rather than the experience itself. For example, Danbury (1996) researched two sets of clients from a national bereavement organisation and a hospice, finding that 47 per cent were dissatisfied with the experience. The main theme was that the clients felt 'let down' by the content of their counselling, as areas of sex, belief in the afterlife, culture and spirituality were not addressed.

A study which provides direct insight into the clients' perspectives of counselling, specifically relating the integration of theory to practice (Flatteau Taylor, 2005), was formed from in-depth interviews with ten bereaved people who had received counselling. The respondents provided insight into their experiences of bereavement and their experiences of counselling, which were analysed to determine what did and did not work for them. The themes which emerged are set out below.

The re-telling of clients' experiences of bereavement noted both the impact and ripple effect of death, and every client's reaction was different. All the respondents continued to relate to and communicate with the deceased in a variety of ways, and this experience was very significant to them, sometimes reassuring and supportive, and at other times having an adverse effect on their ongoing lives.

This research explored the content of counselling and through this gained client evaluations and outcomes. Six participants' counselling experiences were described as unsatisfactory, two felt 'it was OK' and two felt it was satisfactory, as it had been supportive and helpful to them in their grief. The 'unsatisfactory' outcome was noted to be due to:

1. Counsellors relating to stage and task theories: in four instances this truly exacerbated the distress experienced by the clients because they felt they didn't fit the model and that they were 'going round the twist'.

2. Clients perceived that counsellors frequently responded to their continuing relationships and communication with the deceased as 'abnormal'. They reported that their sense of presence of the deceased was either interpreted to them in terms of the 'searching' stage of bereavement, or diverted away from. Therefore, clients did not feel that the reality of their experience was being valued or acknowledged.
3. Sessions were prematurely ended: one client said, 'they just cut the sessions', slashing across the air with her arm, 'just because they said I had got through the angry stage, and had reached acceptance . . . I hadn't, so then I found another counsellor'.
4. The clients wanted to talk about the death, their loss, but found that their counsellors took them in different directions: 'It was just a childhood thing she (the counsellor) wanted to talk about . . . I felt she (was) looking under stones where I didn't need to. And I didn't have a choice'.

The rationale for satisfaction among the minority of respondents was:

1. Primarily they found that their counsellor did not explain, or interpret, their experiences but was alongside them, listening wholeheartedly, accepting them and how they were responding.
2. For some, the importance was that their counsellor facilitated an exploration of their whole story, especially the details of the death, in addition to their experience after death including their ongoing relationship with the deceased, however this manifested itself. They valued this support as they learned to put together the pieces of their shattered lives.

In a nutshell, this study demonstrates that the clients who felt dissatisfied with their counselling had perceived their counsellors to be ill at ease with the subjects they presented to them, as they preferred to hold onto specific theoretical approaches, which did not have a 'good enough' fit with their actual experiences.

The findings of this study appear to tie in with a study by Munichin (1974) who notes that working with clients bereaved by death may lead a counsellor to avoid the subject, sometimes (unwittingly) directing them away from the death through the use of other therapeutic issues.

Another study which explored the perspectives of bereaved clients, as well as that of the counsellors was carried out by Weinstein (1997). This research was based in a hospice, and identifies that clients and counsellors had differing ideas about the focus of the counselling sessions and demonstrates different understandings of the depth of empathy and relationship achieved. Forty-five per cent of the clients felt that their counsellor could empathise with them, whereas 75 per cent of the counsellors felt that they were being empathic.

This shows us the importance of the client leading the sessions; when someone has died the foremost important issue for the client is that the counsellor can step into their shoes, empathise and encourage them to talk about the person, their death, and how life is for them without the deceased.

Research at another hospice-provided bereavement service (Flatteau Taylor and Kuy Kendall, 2009) was carried out with both counsellors and clients. The clients were invited to evaluate their counselling through questionnaire and also through interview. The clients' written evaluations of the service were very positive; however, in the semi-structured interviews some pertinent issues were raised. They noted that they had not known what to expect from counselling and, overall, their positivity reflected their amazement that anyone would be able to support them in their grief. Other comments noted a lack of boundaries for their sessions in timing, and found the counsellors to be quite prescriptive in the way they supported them. They noted that counsellors described to them the stage they were at, and when counselling should end. There tended to be a focus on the collection of memories of the deceased through the use of scrapbooks and memory boxes.

Voices

One client noted:

> *'. . . I made a memory box, it was filled with things, it's nice to keep, but I'll never forget her. I'll always remember her in my own way . . . my counsellor just wanted me to be doing something.'*

Moira

The additional feedback from staff through interviews about their role was very positive and enthusiastic; however, the majority expressed a level of reservation. For example, they identified training as holding an insufficient focus on the issues of death and bereavement, self-awareness and counselling skills. They were also concerned, as some of their clients became very low, that potential suicide risk was 'not touched on'.

This appears to demonstrate the incorporation of theories such as those promoting the recollection of, and relationship to, the deceased (Walter, 1999). However, they are integrated in quite a prescriptive manner in counselling clients. We can also see how evaluation is useful, but to be effective a client needs to know what to expect, in order to evaluate what they have received, and additional insight can be provided through research interviews.

A further study of bereaved clients linked to a hospice (Wilson, 2008) concluded that the counsellors focused solely on the actual facts of their client's bereavement (as noted by the clients) without acknowledging that the death had affected everything. In common with the earlier study, they also noted the high level of importance placed on memorialisation of the deceased. The clients emphasised the fact that they had their memories, continuing relationships with their child and did not need further ways to keep them in their thoughts. The study conclusions identified that the key theories integrated into the counsellors' practice were stages, phases, tasks, the dual process model and continuing bonds (Wilson, 2008).

This reflects Jordan's findings that the counsellors were holding to specific theories, rather than really responding to the needs of their bereaved clients.

The findings of a study of clients facing loss through the illness/disability and/or death of their child (Flatteau Taylor, 2003) outlined some issues for clients but focused on what clients needed and wanted from counselling; notably, this was about a counsellor who was demonstrably able to:

- stay with their story; be with them; step into their world and understand
- listen to whatever they described without deflection without overlaying theories on them; with an 'open heart'
- accept them however they are, whatever views/emotions they want to express
- and yet at times demonstrate an initial understanding by introducing some 'common' feelings when people face loss; normalising yet not prescribing their experiences and helping them in making some sense of a nonsensical world.

Clients outlined that in this way they could grow to accept themselves in their new 'normal'. This ties in with the finding of Jordan and Neimeyer (2003) who note that when 'grief counselling' is provided, the most important element of bereavement interventions will be meeting with someone who is a compassionate, empathic, understanding caregiver (Larson and Hoyt, 2007).

The participants also noted what they wanted from the service itself, specifically that it be well signposted, easily accessible, flexible, and ongoing. They suggested privacy, but did not always stress the need for total confidentiality. This has informed the discussion on professional issues in Chapter 7.

This study informs us through enquiry about 'what would be best' rather than 'what has been provided' and, as such, the respondents provided great clarity.

The next section outlines some specific aspects of death just to provide a glimpse of the diversity of death; additional reading in different areas is recommended.

Specific areas of loss: the diversity of death in research

The primary need for the clients in the studies above is that they are truly heard and understood. A lack of knowledge and self-awareness of the diverse nature of death and grief can and will impact upon our abilities as counsellors; and specific reference to the type of death does not appear to be integrated into the mainstream models/theories which are accessed today (see Chapter 3). Therefore, it is important that we gain some knowledge of current research about different types and ways of death, about how people from different cultures and faiths deal with and understand death. The findings above highlight, however, that we use this information as a backdrop to our counselling to inform and not overshadow the unique experiences of our clients.

Below are just a few examples of different types of deaths with brief notes. (See information about further reading at the end of this chapter.)

Traumatic deaths

Studies have noted that traumatic bereavement, such as sudden infant death syndrome, can result in long-lasting psychological upset. It was also noted that following a traumatic death bereaved people experience higher levels of social problems (identity, relationships, interactions in different setting), withdrawal and isolation being a common outcome (Dyregrov and Dyregrov, 1999; Jordan, 2001).

Suicide

McDaid, *et al.* (2008) note that there is a stigma attached to suicide, which can result in heightened emotional reactions, including a sense of rejection. This, in turn, they suggest can lead to difficulties in coping. In addition to the feelings of numbness, shock, disbelief, guilt and anger, there can also be feelings of shame and blame with thoughts of, for example, 'If I had been there this would not have happened'. Suicide brings up strong reactions to the bereaved, in society and potentially in ourselves.

It is important to note that this is just one study and there is a range of perspectives on suicide; the book noted by Wertheimer (1999) in further reading below may be helpful.

Deaths in the military

Changing attitudes to war and therefore military loss are noted to have an impact on experiences of death and bereavement in this area (Rolls and Chowns, 2011). Military deaths are seen mainly as 'crisis deaths', traumatic and violent, somehow expected and yet sudden. These deaths are followed by procedures, which are contrary to civilian deaths, such as repatriation of the body. This is a military practice and changes the experience to a public rather than private family loss. The family may be unlikely to visit the scene of death if it took place abroad. An inquest is essential when the death occurs overseas; the body then becomes owned by the military and the story of what took place may not be clear. Alternatively, if the death occurs in the UK following an injury abroad, there is often little media coverage and no repatriation ceremony; the death is less visible, somehow less important, and potentially disenfranchised (Cohen *et al.*, 2009).

Within each type of death, you can see, even in these extremely short précis of studies, the ripple effect of the death and that sometimes the differences in the effects are obvious, sometimes more subtle.

HIV/AIDS bereavement

Where medicine is involved there can be significant shifts in treatments, resulting in different thinking around a subject. To illustrate this, the diagnosis for someone being HIV positive has quite recently changed from an immediately life-threatening and life-shortening illness to that of a chronic illness, with the subsequent impact of long-term treatments. For clients, recurrent themes will be around loss and impending loss, in line with others facing chronic illness, alongside the impacts of living with the shadow of death. Perreault (2007) noted the responses of bereaved people who are also HIV positive, such as the survivor syndrome, 'They're all dying . . . What is happening? . . . But I'm still here . . . Why am I still here?' There are also issues of loss around changes in identity and belonging, which were indicated by questions such as 'Who am I now?' and 'Where do I belong?'

This highlights how both the concurrent and future losses of our clients will impact on their responses on bereavement.

Death of a child

The death of a child is highlighted by parents as being 'the wrong order', 'the worst death' and 'losing part of themselves' (Malkinson and Bar-Tur, 2005). Wheeler (2001) notes that a total crisis of meaning is often brought about through child death. Rosenblatt (2004) notes that talking in the present tense does not connect to the parents failing to recognise the reality of their child's death; he suggests that this can be explained in terms that they continue to have a relationship with their child.

Studying such texts, highlighting the issues which parents present will help us to reflect not only on the potential impacts on the bereaved parent, but also the potential impacts on ourselves when counselling; for example, what affect may a client's statement that they have faced a death in 'the wrong order' have on us?

Older people in residential settings

A study of death in residential settings was the centre of a study of six residential homes, Last Rights. Within a population whose death is more likely to be expected, the authors identify issues such as informing the family, helping with practical arrangements following the death and working with the faith and belief of the dying person and their relatives. Summing up the need for dealing with death in residential homes, they define openness, good communication, defined guidelines, sharing of issues, not hidden corners, and the qualities required from staff of empathy, warmth and genuineness. This report also speaks about staff who are noted to experience high levels of stress (Counsel and Care, 1995).

This report about the death of an older person suggests that death is 'more likely to be expected'; will this be our expectation when working with someone whose grandparent has died, for example? What could be the impact of society on the bereaved – perhaps a response of 'well she/he had a good innings'?

Bereavement across cultures: faiths and beliefs

Beliefs and assumptions about death and grief exist in every culture and they can provide a way of making sense of death and loss. Cranstom (1987), in Walter (1999), notes that where faith and religion are mutual it can have the effect of drawing the family and friends together in their grief. Alternatively, where faith differs people can draw apart and feel more isolated in their grief (Klass, 1991).

Wikan notes the great contrast in expressions of grief in different cultures. She notes that:

> 'in Egypt the bereaved are encouraged to dwell profusely on their subjective pain in an atmosphere where . . . others also immerse themselves in tragic tales and expressed sorrow . . . in Bali laughter and cheerfulness fill the air while the bereaved are enjoined to contain their sorrow and may be made to feel they commit an injustice to others should they fail to abide by this demand.'
>
> **Wikan, 1990:455**

This highlights how important it is to be aware of the diversity of death, ways of death, and the context in which that death happens – the cuture and belief of the client. It has been noted that counsellors did not facilitate clients in exploring their faith and belief (Flatteau Taylor, 2005).

This is in no way intended to be an exhaustive list of difference and diversity in death; it is a start point, to make us think. The further reading list below includes some useful texts on the different reactions between men and women, different cultures and beliefs on bereavement.

Summary

- Research – rechercher – means always questioning what you see, what you know and what you do; this is inevitably tiring, but challenging, and thus exciting!
- This chapter notes that research is important for us to integrate into and inform our practice; if we do not update our thinking and reading we could

find a shadow is cast – an area which is not acknowledged or explored that lies between the idea of theory and the reality of client work.

- We need to ensure that we do not become 'culture bound', tapping into theories which we understand, without questioning what the client understands.
- To continue to develop as professionals and to provide the best possible services to our clients, it is important that we keep up to date with current trends and new research. It is important for people working with loss to look for specific areas, in order to find studies and findings, to normalise reading in specialist areas and talk to people with additional knowledge and understanding.

Activity

Consider the theories outlined in Chapter 7 and the ongoing research outlined in this chapter.

Where do you feel your practice would 'sit' in the theories and ideas outlined?

If you have not yet started to practise, where do you think your practice will feel more comfortable?

And ask yourself 'Why?' to both of these questions.

Further reading

The list below includes books which outline studies in specific areas of loss and bereavement (the elderly/culture), as well as an additional text on bereavement and loss in general.

Counsel & Care (1995) *Last Rights: A Study of how Death and Dying are Handled in Residential Care and Nursing Homes*. London: Counsel & Care.

Klass, D. (1991) *Parental Grief, Solace and Resolution*. New York: Springer.

Raphael, B. (1983) *The Anatomy of Bereavement*. New York: Basic Books.

Weinstein, J. (1997) *'My Safe Place' A Report on Havering and Brentwood Bereavement Counselling Services*. London: South Bank University.

Wertheimer, A. (1999) *A Special Scar. The Experiences of People Bereaved by Suicide* (5th edn). London, New York: Routledge.

Wikan, U. (1990) *Managing Turbulant Hearts: A Balinese Formula for Living*. Chicago: University of Chicago Press.

Glossary

Information is not knowledge.

Albert Einstein

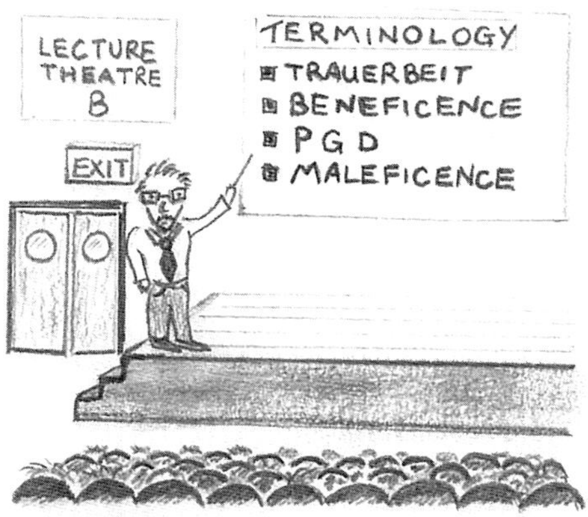

Figure 10.1

This chapter presents a glossary of terms, which gives you information and explanations of terms used to ensure that where we do use specific language, it can be understood and will add to our knowledge base of the subject of loss and bereavement. The subsequent sections note some resources for further study.

Anticipatory grief

refers to a grieving that can sometimes occur before a loss, which may be anticipated. This impending loss can be the death of someone due to illness. It is also said to be experienced by dying individuals themselves.

Autonomy

is the capacity of an individual who is deemed to be able and rational to make an informed, unforced decision. Autonomy is often used as the basis for determining the moral responsibility for one's actions in moral and political philosophy. It is used here to refer to an ethical tenet of the ability to counsel clients to govern themselves.

Beneficence

refers to actions that will do, or produce, good including the promotion of the well being of others. In a medical context, this means taking actions that serve the best interests of patients.

Bereavement

the state of being we are in when we are deprived or something or someone, i.e. following a significant loss (in contemporary society). The forerunner of our modern word 'bereavement' was the old English word bereafian, which included the definitions 'to be robbed' or 'deprived of something valuable'.

Bereavement counselling

in general terms, used to describe a form of counselling that focuses on helping people to cope with grief and mourning following a significant loss, including the death of loved ones, or with major life changes that trigger feelings of grief (e.g., divorce). (Also referred to as grief counselling.)

However, the definition and 'job description' for someone carrying out 'bereavement counselling' are varied. See also Counselling bereaved people below.

Bereavement process

the process we go through when we grieve following a loss is a personal and individual experience; no two people's pathways through grief will be the same. The process has been described in different ways through theories which can be noted in Chapter 3. However, the important factor to note is that there are few 'norms' in grief, no timetable and no specific way 'to do it'. It is important that counsellors are trained to listen to their client's story with an 'open heart' without overlaying theories, and stay alongside them as their story is told and their feelings unfold.

Cognitive behavioural therapy (CBT)

is based on the belief that behaviour is learnt in response to past experience. As such, we can recondition ourselves or unlearn the behaviours without the need to analyse past experiences, to find the reasons or triggers for such behaviours. It is noted to work well for compulsive and obsessive behaviour, fears, phobias and addictions.

Complex medical needs

an illness or disability: where the diagnosis may mean that life is threatened, but the illness may be curable; where the diagnosis means that life will be shortened; where an illness or disability means constant ongoing treatments; may be acquired, i.e. through accident and life may be threatened through surgery or the remaining disability.

Complicated grief

now referred to as prolonged grief disorder (PGD) is a pathological reaction to loss (formerly known as complicated grief). An attempt is being made to create a diagnosis category for complicated grief in the Diagnostic Statistical Manual V (DSM-V); critics of doing so say that it will constitute characterising a natural response as a pathology, and will result in wholesale medicating of people who may otherwise be deemed 'normal' in their grief. This is an area into which I would urge further reading. See also pathological grief.

Confidentiality

requires providers of bereavement support to respect the privacy of each bereaved person and information shared by them. It is essential that the relationship between each bereaved person (the bereaved client) and the individual or agency which offers them support is one of trust. Providers of support to bereaved people in the UK respect the confidentiality and privacy of those who use their service.

The duty to maintain confidentiality extends to all those involved in offering support, including management committees, and continues after that support has stopped and beyond the death of a bereaved client. Confidentiality is not absolute. In exceptional circumstances, it may be necessary to share information about a bereaved client with a third party. This can happen if: the law requires it; there is a real and serious risk of danger or harm to the bereaved client or another person; there has been unethical or criminal behaviour.

Bereaved clients need to be made aware of the limits to confidentiality as soon as possible, preferably before support begins. If information is to be disclosed to a third party, bereaved clients should, wherever possible, give informed and meaningful consent. Any decision to break confidentiality should be discussed with a supervisor or senior colleague before any action is taken. (See UK Bereavement Standards below.)

Counselling bereaved people

help a bereaved person to work through grief in their own way, at their own pace and in their own time; without a specific way to experience bereavement. This book encourages the integration of a 'whole of life' or holistic approach to counselling people on bereavement; therefore, for the purposes of this text the phrase 'counselling for bereaved people' is the preferred term.

Disenfranchise
to deprive of a franchise, of a legal right, or of some privilege or of a franchise in the context of grief (see below).

Disenfranchised grief
a term describing grief that is not acknowledged by society. Examples of grief becoming disenfranchised are: the loss of a pet; a trauma in the family in an earlier generation; the loss of a home or place of residence; an aborted/miscarried pregnancy; a mother's loss or adoption; the death from socially unacceptable causes such as suicide; the death of a celebrity; loss or severe disability of a parent during wartime (others around the child's family may not be able to relate to or support properly).

Disenfranchisement
can also occur when a loss is associated with what is seen as a positive life event: the areas are huge; for example, a marriage when the newly weds may also be leaving home; a graduation, when the graduate is leaving the safety of the university/college and heading to the world of work. Even widely recognised forms of grief can become disenfranchised, when well-meaning friends and family attempt to set a time limit on a bereaved person's right to grieve.

Ethics
a set of principles of right and appropriate conduct and/or a system of moral values. Ethics also includes the study of the general nature of morals and the specific moral choices to be made by a person: moral philosophy. Most importantly, ethics refer to the rules or standards governing the conduct of a person or the members of a profession, such as counselling.

Grief
primarily an emotional reaction to a significant loss; this may be caused by the death of someone close. It will be expressed in many ways: emotionally, behaviourally and physically.

Grief work
the 'work' we do when we grieve can be described as the cognitive process of confronting the loss, of going over the events before and at the time of death, of focusing on memories and working toward detachment from the deceased. It is often associated with the need to create an active, ongoing, effortful attempt to come to terms with loss. This is discussed in the text in terms of the lack of resolution of grief, and need to continue relationships with the deceased (see also Continuing

bonds). (Also named 'Trauerbeit': Freud 1917.) See also Bereavement process.

Holistic

the root of the word holism is ὅλος (holos) – a Greek word meaning all, whole, entire, total; the idea that all aspects of a given cannot be determined or explained by its component parts.

Informed consent

usually refers to the idea that a person must be fully informed about and understand the potential benefits and risks of their choice of treatment. An uninformed person is at risk of mistakenly making a choice that does not reflect his or her values or wishes. It does not specifically mean the process of obtaining consent, nor the specific legal requirements, which vary from place to place for capacity to consent. Patients can elect to make their own medical decisions, or can delegate decision-making authority to another party. If the patient is incapacitated, laws around the world designate different processes for obtaining informed consent; typically a person appointed by the patient, or his or her next of kin, makes decisions for the patient. The value of informed consent is closely related to the values of autonomy and truth telling.

Moral

the lesson or principle contained in, or taught by, a fable, a story, or an event; a concisely expressed precept or general truth; a maxim. Morals are rules or habits of conduct, especially of sexual conduct, with reference to standards of right and wrong: for example, a person of loose morals; a decline in the public morals.

Mourning

as contrasting with grief, is the social expression or acts expressive of grief that are shaped by the practices of a given society or cultural group.

Mutual help group – self-help group

a group of people who provide mutual support for each other. The members will share a common issue or problem; for example, bereavement, or a specific bereavement such as death of a child. The Compassionate Friends provides support based on self-help groups. The goal will be to help each other to deal with this problem through a mutuality of understanding.

Non-maleficence

the first concept is primum non nocere (Latin) 'first, do no harm', referring to the first line of importance not to do harm to your client.

Parallel process

the idea encapsulated through the way in which elements of the counselling relationship can be paralleled to other aspects of life. For example, a client/counsellor relationship may 'parallel' a relationship the client has with other people in his or her life, where certain key aspects of patterns of relating are mirrored.

Pathological grief

Margaret Stroebe (2000) acknowledges that grief can become complicated and, therefore in her view, 'pathological'. However, she suggests that there are no clear guidelines available to establish at what intensity, and/or duration, and/or type of symptomatology grief can be considered pathological. Nor is it evident precisely where and how pathological grief should be placed in a diagnostic system. See also Complicated grief.

Person centred therapy or counselling

can also be named 'client-centred' or 'Rogerian' counselling. It is based on the view that people will, given the right environment, find their own way forward. Through counselling, the 'right environment' will be that of an accepting, genuine, understanding relationship provided by the counsellor. Within this, the client will be able to talk about his or her experiences, express emotions, explore his or her behaviours and develop the resources, in order to make any changes that he or she feels they need to make.

Somatise

to express psychological issues or conflicts through somatic symptoms; people who are bereaved, who feel unable to fully express their feelings, often have chest pains and suffer from a 'broken heart'. This should be medically checked, but when unexplainable by a doctor, could be a somatic symptom of their grief.

Specialist

in this text is as person who devotes himself or herself to one subject, or to one particular branch of a subject or pursuit.

Specialist organisation

can be defined because it has a client group that need special training to understand their needs; in the context of this book, this will be bereaved people. And their client group will require professional qualifications/ specific experience of the staff specific to the area.

Statutory services
are services required to exist by law, e.g. social services and the National Health Service. All local authorities are obliged to provide statutory services, which tend to be those considered as so essential to modern life that for moral reasons their universal provision should be guaranteed.

Trauma
a serious injury or shock to the body, as from violence or an accident; an emotional wound or shock that creates substantial, lasting damage to the psychological development of a person, often leading to neurosis; or an event or situation that causes great distress and disruption.

Unresolved grief (or delayed grief)
any aspect of grieving that has yet to be resolved. In cases of unresolved or delayed grief, the reaction to the loss is postponed until a later time, even years later, and might be triggered by a seemingly unrelated event, such as a recent divorce or even the death of a pet, but with reactions that are excessive to the current situation. The resolution of grief is sometimes indefinable, and occurrences of repeated expressions of grief can be a normal response to a new, even unrelated, experience of loss.

Vicarious traumatisation
a term coined with specific reference to counselling and therapists who work with clients who survive trauma. Resulting from being empathic with traumatised clients, therapists will be changed in their sense of meaning of the world and life experiences.

Voluntary service
an organisation that undertakes voluntary activities, i.e. those which do not have to be provided by law (statutory services). They have the following additional characteristics: clear objectives, contents and tasks, structure and framework, appropriate support.

Volunteers/voluntary activities
have the following characteristics: open to all, unpaid, undertaken of own free will, educational (non-formal learning aspect), adding social value.

References

ACT/RCPCH (1997) *A Guide to the Development of Children's Palliative Care Services*. London: ACT and RCPCH.

ACT/RCPCH (2003), *A Guide to the Development of Children's Palliative Care Services*. 2nd edn, Bristol: ACT/RCPCH.

ACT CARE PATHWAY 2003b, Soutter *et al.*, 1994; Beresford, 1995; While *et al.*, 1996a; Putt and McElhill, 1995; Dobson and Middleton, 1998; Dobson *et al.*, 2001; Corden *et al.*, 2001.

Ainsworth, M. D. S. and Bell, S. M. (1970) 'Attachment, exploration, and separation: Illustrated by the behavior of one-year-olds in a strange situation', *Child Development*, 41, 49–67.

Amis, K. (2008) 'Working with Client Dependency', in Dryden, W and Reeves, A. *Key Issues for Counselling in Action*, 2nd edn. London: Sage (172–82).

Aries, P. (1981) *The Hour of Our Death*. London: Penguin.

Attig, T. (1996) *How We Grieve: Relearning the World*. Oxford: Oxford University Press.

Bond, T. (2000) *Standards and Ethics for Counselling in Action* (Counselling in Action series). London: Sage.

Bowlby, J. (1969–1980) *Attachment and Loss*, Volumes 1–3. New York: Basic Books.

Bowlby, J. and Parkes, C.M. (1970) 'Separation and loss within the family' in E.J. Anthony and C. Koupernik (eds) *The Child in his Family, International Yearbook of Child Psychiatry and Allied Professionals* Vol 1. New York: John Wiley.

Bowlby, J. (1979) *The Making and Breaking of Affectional Bonds*. London: Tavistock.

British Association for Counselling and Psychotherapy (2010) *Ethical Framework for Good Practice in Counselling & Psychotherapy*. Lutterworth: BACP.

Brooks, D. (1997) *Beat Stress from Within*. Minneapolis: Hollanden.

Cambridge Advanced Learner's Dictionary & Thesaurus. Cambridge: Cambridge University Press.

Carmichael, J. (in press, 2013) *Challenges for Counsellors: Research*. London: Hodder Stoughton.

Centre for Grief Education (2001) Minimum Standards for the Provision of Support Programmes in Palliative Care Services in Victoria **www.grief.org.au**

Childrens Hospices UK (2011) *Standards framework for children's palliative care*, **www.togetherforshortlives/professional/resources**.

Cohen, J. A., Goodman, R. F., Cambell, C., Caroll, B. L. and Campagna, H. (2009) 'Military children, the sometimes orphan of war', in Freeman Moore and Freeman (eds) *Living and Surviving in Harms Way: A Psychological Treatment Handbook for Pre- and Post-deployment of Military Personnel*. New York: Routledge (395–416).

Coppola, K. M. and Strohmetz, D. B. (2002) 'How is death and dying addressed in introductory psychology textbooks?' *Death Studies* 26, 689–99.

Counsel & Care (1995) *Last Rights: A Study of how Death and Dying are Handled in Residential Care and Nursing Homes*. London: Counsel & Care.

Craib, I. (1994) *The Importance of Disappointment*. London: Routledge.

Danbury, H. (1996) *Bereavement Counselling Effectiveness: A Client Opinion Study*. London: Avebury.

Diagnostic and Statistical Manual of Mental Disorders DSM IV (1994). USA: American Psychiatric Association.

Doka, K. (ed.) (1989) *Disenfranchised Grief: Recognising Hidden Sorrow*. Lexington MA: Lexington Books.

Dryden, W. and Reeves A. (eds) (2008) *Key Issues for Counselling in Action*. London: Sage.

Dyregrov, K., Nordanger, D. and Dyregrov, A. (2003) 'Predictors of psychosocial distress after suicide SIDS and accidents', *Death Studies* 27, 143–65.

Dyregrov, K. and Dyregrov, A. (1999) 'Long term impact of sudden infant death: a twelve to fifteen year follow-up', *Death Studies* 23, 635–61.

Dyregrov, K. (2004) 'Does professional assistance empower or disempower people after traumatic death, *Scandinavian Journal of Psychology* Vol 45.2: 181–189.

Flatteau Taylor, S. and Kuykendall, J. (2009) 'External review of hospice care service for bereavement services', (unpublished).

Flatteau Taylor, S. (2005) 'Between the idea and the reality: study counselling experiences of bereaved people', *Counselling and Psychotherapy Research*, 5(1): 53–61.

Flatteau Taylor, S. (2003) 'Identifying the psychosocial needs of families with children with complex medical needs; The Maypole Project research study', (unpublished).

Flatteau Taylor, S. (2012) 'A notebook for psychosocial support in supporting families with children who have complex medical needs', (unpublished).

Flatteau Taylor, S. (2012) 'Footprint Guide: psychosocial support guideline for children with complex medical needs and their families', (unpublished).

Frankl, V. (1959) *Man's Search for Meaning; the Classic Tribute to Hope in the Holocaust*. London: Ebury.

Freud, S. (1917) 'Mourning and melancholia', in Freud S., (ed) *On Metapsychology*. London: Pelican Freud Library (1st edn 1984).

Fulton, R. (ed) (1965) *Death and Identity*. New York: John Wiley & Sons.

Gorer, G. (1965) *Death, Grief, and Mourning in Contemporary Britain*. London: Cresset Press.

Haugh, S. and Mercy, T. (2001) *Rogers' Therapeutic Conditions*. Ross-on-Wye: PCCS Books.

Haugh, S. (2011) 'A person centred approach to loss and bereavement', in Tolan, J. and Wilkins, P. *Client Issues in Counselling and Psychotherapy*. London: Sage (18–29).

Horowitz, M.J., Siegal, B., Holen, A., Bonanno, G.A., Milbrat, C. and Stinson, C.H. (1997), 'Diagnostic Criteria for complicated grief disorder', *American Journal of Psychiatry*, 154 (904–910)

Jacoby, L. H., Breitkopf, C. R. and Pease, E. A. (2005) 'A qualitative examination of the needs of families faced with the option of organ donation', *Dimensions of Critical Care Nursing*, 24(4): 183–9.

Jordan, J.R. (2000) 'Research that matters: Bridging the gap between research and practice in thematology', *Death Studies.* 24: 6, 457–467.

Jordan, J. R. (2001) 'Is suicide bereavement different? A reassessment of the literature', *Suicide and Life-Threatening Behaviour,* 31, 91–102.

Jordan, J. R. and Neimeyer, R. A. (2003) 'Does grief counselling work?' *Death Studies,* 27: 765–786.

Kirchberg, T. M., Neimeyer, R. A. and James, R. K. (1998) 'Beginning counsellors' death concerns and empathic responses to client situations involving death and grief', *Death Studies,* 22: 99–120.

Klass, D., Silverman P. and Nickman, S. (eds) (1999) *Continuing Bonds: New Understandings of Grief.* Washington DC: Taylor & Francis.

Kübler-Ross, E. (1969) *On Death and Dying.* New York, NY: Simon and Schuster.

Kübler-Ross, E. (1971) *Interviews with the Dying.* Stuttgart: Cross.

Larson, D. and Hoyt, W. T. (2007) 'What has become of grief counseling?', *Professional Psychology Research and Practice,* 38, 4, 347–55.

Lewis, C. S. (2001) *A Grief Observed.* London: HarperOne.

Lindemann, E. (1944) 'Symptomatology and management of acute grief', *American Journal of Psychiatry,* 101: 141–8.

Luft, J. and Ingham, H. (1955) *The Johari Window: a Graphic Model for Interpersonal Relations.* University of California Western Training Lab.

Malkinson, R. and Bar-Tur, L. (2005) 'Long term bereavement processes of older parents; the three phases of grief', *Omega* 50: 103–29.

Martin, T. and Doka, K. (2000) *Men Don't Cry, Women Do: Transcending Gender Stereotypes of Grief.* Philadelphia PA: Brunner Mazel.

McDaid, C., Trowman, R., Golder, S., Hawton, K. and Sowden, A. (2008) 'Interventions for people bereaved through suicide: systematic review', *The British Journal of Psychiatry,* 193: 438–43.

Munichin, R. (1974) in McBride, J. and Simms, S. (2001) 'Death in the family: adapting a family systems framework to the grief process', *The American Journal of Family Therapy,* 29, 1, 59–73.

National Bereavement Consortium Initiative (2001) 'Standards for Bereavement Care in the UK', Bereavement Care Standards UK (unpublished).

National Institute for Health and Clinical Excellence (March, 2004) *Improving Supportive and Palliative Care for Adults with Cancer*. **guidance.nice.org.uk/guidance**

Neimeyer, R. A. (2000) 'Searching for the meaning of meaning: Grief therapy and the process of reconstruction', *Death Studies*, 24: 541–58.

Neimeyer, R.A. (2001) *Lessons of Loss: A Guide to Coping. London*: Brunner Rouledge.

Paulson, B., Everall, R. and Stuart, J. (2001) 'Client perceptions of hindering experiences in counselling', *Counselling and Psychotherapy Research*, 1(1): 53–61.

Perreault, P. (2007) 'The presence of absence: the effect of HIV serostatus on the bereavement experiences of long-term survivors of multiple AIDS-related losses' Royal Roads University Thesis (Accessed on 16.10.12) **www.abrpo.org/images/uploads/Presence%20of%20Absence.pdf**

Powell, J. (1999) *Why Am I Afraid to Tell You Who I Am?* London: Fount.

Prigerson, H.J. (1990) 'Consensus criteria for traumatic grief: a preliminary empirical test' *British Journal of Psychiatry* 174: 67–73.

Rando, T. (1993) *Treatment of Complicated Mourning*. Champaign, IL: Research Press.

Raphael, B. (1983) *Anatomy of Bereavement*. New York: Basic Books.

Reeves, A. (2010) *Counselling Suicidal Clients (Therapy in Practice)*. London: Sage.

Reeves, A., Bowl, R., Wheeler, S. and Guthrie, E. (2004) 'The dialogue of suicide', *Counselling and Psychotherapy Research*, 4, 1.

Resnick, J. (2004) 'The clinical implications of dependency and counter dependency', *Psychotherapy in Australia*, 10(3): 52–9.

Riches, G. and Dawson, P. (2000) *An Intimate Loneliness*. Oxford: OU Press.

Rogers, C. (1951) *Client Centred Therapy: Its Current Implications and theory*. Boston: Houghton Mifflin.

Rogers, C. (1972) *Empathic: An Unappreciated Way of Being.* (Accessed online 2012) **www.elementsuk.com/libraryofarticles/empathic.pdf**

Rolls, L. and Chowns, G. (2011) 'Meeting the needs of those bereaved through military death. Findings from a literature review and scoping study', Commissioned by Forces Support.

Rosenblatt, P. (2001) 'Grief: The social context of private feelings', in M. Stroebe, W. Stroebe and R. Hansson (eds) *Handbook of Bereavement: Theory, Research and Intervention.* Cambridge: Cambridge University Press (102–11).

Rosenblatt, P. (2004) 'Parents talking in the present tense about their dead child', *Bereavement Care* 19, 3, winter 2008, 335–9.

Rowling, L. (2003) *Grief in School Communities: Effective Support Strategies.* Buckingham: OU Press.

Schmid, P. F. (2001a) 'Comprehension: the art of not-knowing. Dialogical and ethical perspectives on empathy as dialogue in personal and person-centred relationships', in Haugh, S. and Merry, T. (eds) Rogers' *Therapeutic Conditions Evolution, Theory and Practice. Volume 2: Empathy.* Ross-on-Wye: PCCS Books (53–71).

Schmid, P. F. (2001b). 'The necessary and sufficient conditions of being person-centered', in Watson, J. *et al.* (eds) *Client-centered and Experiential Psychotherapy in the 21st Century: Advances in Theory, Research and Practice.* Ross-on-Wye: PCCS Books.

Selye, H. (1976) *The Stress of Life* (rev. edn). New York: McGraw-Hill.

Sexton, L. (1999) 'Vicarious traumatisation of counsellors and effects on their workplaces', *British Journal of Guidance and Counselling*, 27, 3.

Stroebe, M., van Son M., Stroebe, W., Kleber R., Schut, H. and van den Bout, J. (2000) 'On the Classification and Diagnosis of pathological grief', *Clinical Psychology Review*, 20, 1, 57–75.

Stroebe, M. and Schut, H. (2005) 'Interventions to enhance adaptation to bereavement', *Journal of Palliative Medicine*, 8, 140–7.

Stroebe, M. (1992) 'Coping with bereavement: a review of the grief work hypothesis', *Omega, Journal of Death and Dying*, 26,19–42.

Stroebe, M., Hansson, R., Stroebe W. and Schut, H. (2001) *Handbook of Bereavement Research: Consequences Coping and Care.* Washington: American Psychological Association.

Stroebe, M., Stroebe, W., Schut, H., van den Bout, J. and Zech, E. (2002) 'Does disclosure of emotions facilitate recovery from bereavement?' *Journal of Consulting and Clinical Psychology*, 70, 1: 169–78.

Stroebe, M. and Schut, H. (1999) 'The dual process model of coping with bereavement: rationale and description', *Death Studies*, 23: 197–224.

Tolan, J. and Wilkins, P. *Client Issues in Counselling and Psychotherapy*. London: Sage (18–29).

Truax, C. B. and Carkhuff, R. R. (1967) *Toward Effective Counselling and Psychotherapy Training and Practice*. Chicago: Aldine-Atherton.

The University of Nottingham (2010) 'Bereavement Care Services: a synthesis of the literature'.

Walter, T. (1991) 'Modern death: taboo or not taboo?' *Sociology*, 25, 2: 293–310.

Walter, T. (1996) 'A new model of grief: bereavement and biography', *Mortality* 1:1: 7–25.

Walter, T. (1999) *On Bereavement: the Culture of Grief*. Buckingham: OU Press.

Weinstein, J. (2002) 'A shoulder to support me, not a shoulder to cry on', South Bank University (unpublished).

Wertheimer, A. (1999) *A Special Scar. The Experiences of People Bereaved by Suicide* (5th edn). London, New York: Routledge.

Wheeler, J. (2001) 'Parental bereavement: the crisis of meaning', *Death Studies*, 25(1): 51–66.

Wilson, G. (2008) 'How effective is provision to support bereaved families within palliative care services' (unpublished).

Worden, J. W. (2008) (1981, 1991 2nd edn) *Grief Counselling and Grief Therapy: A Handbook for the Mental Health Practitioner* (4th edn). New York: Springer.

Yalom, I. (1989) *Love's Executioner and Other Tales of Psychotherapy*. London: Penguin.

Appendix: resources for further study

This section is a brief list and is not exhaustive. It provides an idea of the guidelines available. Please check with your local services for other standards available.

Standards and guidelines for loss and bereavement

While there are many local standards, the national guidelines include those set out below.

National Institute for Health and Clinical Excellence

Outlines three level components of bereavement support:

- level 1: grief is normal, at this level most people manage without professional intervention.
- level 2: support may be required, but this will probably be informal, befrienders, self-help groups, etc.; there needs to be a clear referral process here to level 3 (see below) in cases where complex issues emerge.
- level 3: a minority of people require specialist interventions: specialist counselling, psychotherapy, bereavement services, psychological support, mental health services.

UK Bereavement Standards

Created in 2001, the UK Bereavement Standards are aimed primarily at the voluntary sector, as 80 per cent of bereavement support is defined as being delivered by voluntary services. It is also defined as a 'work in progress'; unfortunately, the council that was proposed to continue to develop these standards and to monitor any services that adopted them was not created.

They advocate services which promote grief as a natural experience, and that services should be responsive, non-discriminatory and confidential. To this end they should have policies and procedures in place to ensure that they provide adequate information about the services they provide, its boundaries, and staff who are adequately trained and supervised, with adequate monitoring and evaluation in place.

Guidelines for best practice in a children's hospice (Children's Hospices UK, 2011)

Outlines:

- ongoing support to be integral to the care of the family
- respectful of culture and religious needs
- can continue as long as is necessary; with negotiated ending
- supervision/support for staff essential
- skills and experience essential, as is working with other agencies who may also be working with the family.

www.togetherforshortlives/professionals/resources

The Maypole Project 'Footprint Guide'

Unpublished, available from: The Maypole Project, 51 High Street, Green Street Green

BR6 6BQ

01689 851596.

info@themaypoleproject.co.uk

www.themaypoleproject.co.uk

Courses

The following organisations offer courses specialising in loss; again, search for the plethora of courses which will be available in your locality.

Child Bereavement UK

The Saunderton Estate, Wycombe Road, Saunderton, Buckinghamshire HP14 4BF

Tel: 01494 568900

www.childbereavement.org.uk

Providing: training, support and information for professionals and families.

Help the Hospices & St Christophers

St Christopher's Hospice, 51–59 Lawrie Park Road, Sydenham, London SE26 6DZ

Tel: 020 8768 4500

info@stchristophers.org.uk

www.stchristophers.org.uk/education

Providing: a full range of education programmes from medical to psycho social.

Laces: loss across consultancy, education, support

51 High Street, Green Street Green, Orpington BR6 6BQ

Tel: 01689 889 880

www.laces-support.co.uk

Providing: training in loss and bereavement; workshops/bespoke training/ university accredited course; also specialist supervision, consultancy.

The Maypole Project

51 High Street, Green Street Green, Orpington BR6 6BQ

Tel: 01689 851596

Providing: training in all aspects of loss and bereavement, including supporting families facing loss when a child is diagnosed with a chronic illness or disability.

Examples of specialist journals

Mortality
Available at: **www.tandfonline.com/toc/cmrt20/current**

Death Studies
Available at: **www.tandfonline.com/toc/udst20/current**

Omega: Journal of Death and Dying
Available at: **baywood.com/journals/previewjournals.asp?id=0030**

Cruse *Bereavement Care* journal
Available at: **www.crusebereavementcare.org.uk/BCJournal.html**

Paedpallit – provides abstracts of research about children's palliative care.

Available at: **www.togetherforshortlives.org.uk/professionals/service_planning/research_abstracts**

Research centre re. death

Centre for Death & Society, Department of Social & Policy Sciences, University of Bath, Bath BA2 7AY

Tel: 01225 386949

Email: **cdas@bath.ac.uk**

Index

Page numbers in italics indicate diagrams; pages numbers bold indicate a glossary entry.